COMAVILLE

KEVIN BIGLEY

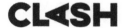

CL◢SH

"I'd trade all of my tomorrows for just one single yesterday."

JENNY LOU CARSON

CHAPTER ONE

JOSH HUSK AWOKE IN A BED THAT HAD ONCE BELONGED to him. The sun peered through the nearby window, gently stroking his face. He lay there for a brief moment, feeling the textures enveloping him. The bed was much too small for him, his legs dangling over the side at mid-shin. He sat up, confused and alert as if he had just left a nightmare behind. He took in the room. It was foreign, yet familiar.

The floor was a sprawling, orange, shag carpet; a disgusting sea of burnt pumpkin. Sparse blotches of brown were mixed in, which seemed more like accidents than artistic choices. The length of the shag bordered on experimental, reaching almost two inches in height.

A dial television set sat on the floor, surrounded by an old gaming console. The controllers sat amongst the shag, their wires tangled in unsolvable knots, snaking through the carpet. Action figures were scattered about like the bodies of fallen soldiers. The walls were blanketed with posters from Saturday morning cartoons and beloved video game characters.

It became apparent to Josh, at that moment, that this was his childhood bedroom.

He was thirty-six-years old, but was somehow sitting in a room from his childhood; from when he was ten, to be exact. Josh had moved around as a kid, his father being a drill sergeant in the military. He had collected an assortment of childhood bedrooms, but this one had always loomed large in his memory. There was a large oak tree resting just outside his window. It managed to block the sun on summer days, allowing him to sleep in late, while also providing autumnal bursts of color as the seasons changed. The shag carpet, although hideous, served as an added cushion for rough-housing, protecting him and his friends from unexpected adventures to the ER. And the walnut wood paneling gave the room the warmth of an old den, like that of an intellectual. It used to make Josh feel older than he was.

He examined the sheets and remembered them immediately. They were the very same sheets his grandmother had given him for Christmas last year. Well, not last year. When he was nine, actually.

Why am I here, he thought. And why am I wearing my fancy jammies?

These were a pair of royal blue pajamas, made up of artificial silk. They were his favorite pair. His mother used to call them his "fancy jammies" because he looked like a young gentleman when he wore them. They even came with a bubble pipe that he would smoke while he read his comic books.

"Welp," he'd say, gently closing the adventures of some caped crusader. "Time to turn in." It always got a big laugh from his parents.

But these fancy jammies had obviously been modified to fit a thirty-six-year-old man.

And speaking of his parents: he couldn't remember them. He knew he had them, a mother and father, he even recalled the places they'd lived and some of the things they'd done as a unit: trips, excursions, routines, etc. He vaguely remembered arguments and lectures, perhaps even a funny anecdote they had said or done, but a mental barrier had been erected in his skull that kept him from tangible remembrance. Their faces, shapes, and voices were absent from even the furthest reaches of his brain. Who were they? What were they like? Did he have siblings? Cousins? Aunts and Uncles? Yes, he knew he had a family. But he could only feel the vague, natural idea of them, the personal specifics being muddied by a blanket of fog, only the shadows of episodes and locations becoming clear in fleeting flashes that lurched at him abruptly and vanished as quickly as they had appeared.

He stood, bewildered and overwhelmed. He hadn't been able to close his hanging jaw since he realized where he was. He felt compelled to explore the rest of the house.

He opened the bedroom door, which revealed a hallway. He carefully entered the dark hall where he found photos hanging from the shadowed walls. The mental fog lingered, like that of a severe hangover, which was only compounded by the peculiar nature of the pictures housed within the frames. They were of Josh at various ages, enjoying various stages of his life, but he couldn't quite remember them. His first trip to a famous theme park, the time he made the twelve-year-old little league all-stars, his eighth-grade graduation, homecoming. He recognized them, but only vaguely. There were also glaring omissions. He was alone in almost all of them. It was as if people had vanished from the pictures, or been physically removed, leaving Josh by himself. In some, he had his arms draped around nothingness, the frame of the photo naturally too large for a self-portrait.

The hallway led into the kitchen where the rest of the house could be seen. This house was not the house he remembered. This was a house unlike any house he had ever lived in because every room belonged to a different stage of his life. And they were seamlessly stitched together. The kitchen was the same kitchen his family had renovated when they had moved to Oregon. The living room was the living room from their house in Evanston. Through a sliding glass door, Josh could see the backyard, which was the same back yard he and his roommates from college had thrown many a summer bbq during his time at the University of Chicago. It was a Frankensteined home of memory. Josh stood, gorgonized and incapable of movement.

"Hello?" Josh called out to no one in particular.

His gaze was drawn to the dining room table, upon which sat a sacked lunch with a post-it note pasted onto it. He approached the bag, picking up the note, which had been impetuously scrawled in red sharpie.

"Have a nice day at work ;)"

While dumbstruck, Josh felt compelled to normalize his situation. If this were a dream, he would inevitably wake from it. And from what he could surmise, he had a job to do.

He showered in the bathroom that once belonged to his family when they had lived in San Diego. It was his favorite shower as it had a detachable head with a massage setting. In his bedroom, he opened the closet to find only one available outfit hanging: a flashy, blue suit. It was the exact suit he had worn to his uncle's wedding. He was eleven-years-old. He had been convinced that he was fully capable of picking out a suit of his own. After persistent badgering, his parents finally caved. He had settled on a gaudy, blue suit with flecks of glitter stitched into the fabric of the pants and coat.

"What a dapper young man," all of the adults had said, laughing to one another.

Josh, being unable to pick up on their subtlety, had thrown a look to his parents, as if to say, "Told ya."

After adorning the suit, he stared into the mirror. It was tailored to perfection. He felt a lump in his right pocket. As he thrust his hand in, he felt the unmistakable shape of car keys. He grabbed his sacked lunch and headed for the door.

The front lawn was the lawn from his family's Evanston home. It was his favorite lawn as there was a large elm on the front of the property, from which hung the tire swing he had made when he was thirteen.

"Hey, Joshua!" a voice cried from next door.

Josh turned, frightened. There, working on his lawn mower, was George Pennygrove; his old Evanston neighbor. George was always friendly, an enthusiastic charmer who built model airplanes in his garage. Josh had often helped him with their assembly, marveling at Pennygrove's craftsmanship and many planes fastened to the walls and rafters.

"...hey, Mr. Pennygrove..."

"If you have some time after work, I'm working on a B-29 bomber. She's shaping up to be a real beauty. You should come by."

"Oh. Okay, Mr. Pennygrove."

"Love the suit, pal. Lookin' sharp. Very dapper."

With that, George's lawn mower roared to life. Josh stood and watched him for a moment, amazed by the familiarity. He took in the street, which was much different from what he remembered. That was because, similar to the inside of his house, it was an amalgamation of streets he had lived on. Across from him sat the Graham's house, home to Steve Graham, whom Josh went to elementary school with. Next to the Grahams was the two-story home of Patty Miller, who babysat Josh when his parents had worked late. Darryl Herb, the friendly dean of his alma-mater, lived down the street. Weirder still, a house over from George's was a fictional house: the house from his favorite sitcom. He couldn't remember the name, but it was that one about the wealthy family who had a poor nephew who came to live with them, and boy did he liven things up! Next to that house sat a massive, plain, birdhouse. It was the exact birdhouse that Josh had built in shop class in the seventh grade. It loomed as large as any house on the block. The street was lined with beloved homes from memory, from television, and from imagination.

A chill went down Josh's spine as he looked towards the driveway and found the car of his dreams. It was a much larger version of a toy car he had owned when he was a boy. It was a 1957 Cadillac Coupe Deville. The car was candy apple red with white-wall tires, large fins with white and red tail lights, and a thick layer of wax that made it sparkle. It was an illustrious work of art.

Josh popped the key into the door, turning it slowly. It opened. He carefully slid into the driver's seat, as if he were being pulled inside by a manipulative lover. The steering wheel was oversized and polished, resting firmly in his grasp. He put the key into the ignition and brought the masterpiece to life. It purred with American muscle and capability, eagerly awaiting Josh's instructions.

He put the Coupe in reverse, gently backing out of the driveway. The car drove like a boat, puttering forward with ease. He could feel it burning a museum's worth of dinosaurs as it hovered above the perfectly paved blacktop. As he drifted down the street, a breeze brushed his chestnut hair, caressing his face. Neighbors, old friends, teachers, familiar television actors, human-sized birds from the birdhouse, all ventured onto their lawns to witness Josh driving past in his chariot. They offered up salutary waves to him as if he were leading an invisible parade. He captained his ship, wading through a sea of jovial worshipers.

Josh relaxed his shoulders, letting all doubt and confusion slip away. Wherever he was, he was welcome. An internal warmth burned inside of him as an easy smile crept across his face. As he turned onto another avenue, it quickly became a highway. Smooth, straight, and empty. Josh accelerated, feeling the power glide the dream car towards the horizon. In the distance, Josh saw a city. It shined like a beacon, its many nitid windows and structures reflecting the iridescent light like a free-standing surface of water. Josh felt the urge to hurtle towards it. He was unsure of the destination, but it gave him the feeling of home. His foot pressed further onto the rumbling gas pedal, pushing the car to its welcomed limits as the wind brushed his scalp with the gentle caress of a loved one.

CHAPTER TWO

STEPHANIE CARESSED HER OLDER BROTHER'S HEAD WITH the tenderness of a random street patron attempting to comfort a frail, recalcitrant animal. She felt great worry for him, terrified that he'd break into pieces if she so much as touched him too coarsely.

Josh had been hit while riding his bike to work, zooming through a parlous intersection where many accidents had occurred before. However, they had usually been of the car-on-car variety. Ever the perpetual child, Josh had obdurately refused to heed Stephanie's warning of wearing a helmet and obeying simple traffic laws, so he had sped through the intersection, witnesses saying he ignored the stop sign, failing to acknowledge the oncoming car until it was too late.

Such a child, Steph thought as she surveyed her brother's bruised skin. Hideous bumps and blossoming bruises littered his body. His eye sockets were a deep purple, the surface of his forehead scratched with crimson red. It was disturbing to see a man usually so filled with ebullient joy being reduced to an unconscious mess.

Steph despised hospitals. Their mother had worked in them all their life. The family had moved around with their father's military career, so they'd seen many different ones, but to Steph, they were all the same. They were filled with the sick, anyone and everyone wishing they weren't where they were. The sterile miasma of foreign chemicals invaded her nostrils. And the artwork was always exceptionally terrible. Watercolors of ships in harbors, rolling fields of listless picnickers, or some bucolic setting and a quaint cottage in the middle of nowhere. Each room had blinding, alabaster walls with the occasional trim of pastel colors. The atmosphere, like the art, was devoid of feeling, opinion, or emotion, as if this were a tactic to quash any feelings of panic or despair. They were blank canvases, assuring that anything that was projected was a result of your personal thought and experience. Both the miraculous and the tragic could unfold. The unbelievable recovery as well as the obligatory turn-for-the-worse. They were scales of fortune, teetering towards results devoid of all reason. She fucking hated hospitals.

She had received the call at work.

"Is this Stephanie Husk?"

"Yes. Well, Stephanie Koehler-Husk. But yes, it is. May I ask who-"

"I'm sorry, Ms. Husk, but I'm calling from St. Joseph's. Your brother, Josh, has been hit by a car. He's stable but unconscious at the moment. You should probably come down here as soon as possible."

"Oh... oh my god."

"He's stable. Like I said, you should get here as soon as you can."

"Sure. Sure. Yes... by a car? Was he riding his bike?"

"He's at St. Joseph's, so just get here as soon as you can and we can fill you in."

Steph was the emergency contact, which was bound to piss her mother off.

Doctor Kaspin entered the room with the phlegmatic rote of a man who was constantly prepared for the scales to tip in either direction. He had committed to his balding scalp, which Steph liked immediately because it showed he was pragmatic. He pulsed with a palpable aura of capability. He was a doctor from the 1960s who probably didn't put any stock in holistic medicine or nonphysical therapy. He surveyed Josh's chart, barely taking the time to look Steph in the eye.

"Hello, I'm Dr. Kaspin. Are you Mrs. Husk? Perhaps the spouse?"

"I am Mrs. Husk, the sister. Mrs. Koehler-Husk. He does not have a spouse."

"Well, let me tell you where we're at. As you can see, he's breathing on his own which is very good. However, I have had the nurses attempt various stimuli, which he is not responding to. And that is not very good."

"Uh huh."

"Now that's not to say that things can't change. They can, for better or worse. Head injuries are a tricky thing because we often don't know their severity until days, sometimes weeks afterward. We need to do a CAT scan so we can evaluate how much damage the brain underwent during his accident. We'll also need to schedule an MRI, which will give us a better look at the brain, but also its functionality. These things, head injuries I mean, are touch and go. A lot can change in twenty-four hours, so we need to keep him closely monitored, make sure there's no bleeding, things like that. But for right now, he's stable, which is good."

Steph had a distant look. Dr. Kaspin noticed.

"I know this is a lot, Mrs. Husk."

"Yes," she said, snapping to. "Sorry, it's just that my mother is going to want to hear all of this. She should be here very soon."

With that, a flurry of scudding footsteps was heard as the hurried gait flew into the room. Lisa and Rich Husk were now present.

"Thank god. Oh thank god we made it," said Lisa skirting between Steph and Dr. Kaspin to Josh's side. "Oh my god. My baby. Oh, my poor baby." She gingerly caressed his bruised and battered face, an inveterate cosseter to her beloved boy.

Lisa Husk was a thin, one could almost say gaunt, woman. She wore her early sixties like hardened armor, making her a sprightly, fierce force to be reckoned with. As long as Steph could remember, her mother had only worn earth tones. She had recently switched to blacks; she wore black galoshes, a long, black skirt, and a dark blouse with sleeves that stretched to her wrists. She carried with her an obsequious air, haughty and reserved. She had piercing blue eyes that shone like sparkling costume jewelry. Her hair was shoulder-length with the coarse, grey look of steel wool. Warmth did not come easily to her, of course with the exception of her baby boy.

"What is his status? What is your plan?" she pushed.

"They want to do a CAT scan," said Steph.

"I was asking the doctor, dear," Lisa hissed. Steph retreated, folding her arms and rolling her eyes.

"Now let's just try to calm down," said Rich. Lisa slowly turned to him, offering her icy eyes, leering at him with severe reprobation. He had misstepped and knew it.

Rich Husk was tall and fit, standing at a lean 6'3". He wore straight-fit khakis and comfortable running shoes with a tucked in polo. In the summers it was the same outfit, except shorts. He was a man who was prepared to golf at a moment's notice. Although his muscles had begun to break apart, his athletic frame was still intact. He had run four marathons after the age of fifty-three and had recently completed a full Iron Man. Although his chiseled jaw and crewcut sent the message of a hard-wired military man, Rich was precisely the opposite. He was as soft as table butter: a notorious cryer at movies, and recently, a man who loved to partake in a long hug. Steph had noticed her father becoming more vulnerable with age, a sweetheart of sweethearts.

"What's his Glasgow Rating?" asked Lisa, aggressive in her quizzing of the doctor. She had only recently retired from her life-long medical career. She still volunteered on weekends.

Dr. Kaspin was surprised by her gumption. "That's difficult to determine without an MRI, Mrs. Husk."

"I don't think we'll be doing that, Doctor. We'll be moving him to my hospital."

Rich touched her shoulder, but Lisa brushed it off like an anxious quarter horse.

"I don't recommend that," said Dr. Kaspin.

"Does he have any blocked arteries? What's in his IV? Are we giving him nutrients? What's the percentage of consciousness?"

"Again, we don't know yet. And I'm assuming, Mrs. Husk, you know that we don't know that."

She scoffed. "We're moving him to Holy Cross. End of story."

"Mom," said Steph. "I think we should listen to Dr. Kaspin."

"Look, I don't have time to debate someone who has already made up their mind," said Dr. Kaspin. "He's your son, but I highly recommend that you do not move him. I'm very confident in my staff and the plan we have in place. We can have an MRI done in the next two hours."

Lisa's cold gaze softened as it moved to her son. The ferocity returned as she brought it back to the doctor. She gave him a slight nod. Dr. Kaspin received the gesture as his opportunity to leave and quickly slid out the door.

"I've never met a doctor who was gifted in communication, and he is no exception," said Lisa.

"So, we're not moving him?" asked Rich.

"Of course not," she said. "We just want to give them the impression that we're not afraid to move him. They want him here. Brain injuries call for extensive tests, which leads to lots of insurance money. We want to put the pressure on them so they make him as much of a priority as possible." She fluffed Josh's pillow. "These pillows are terrible. And whoever put in this IV needs to go back to school. I'm going to find his nurse and make a few things clear."

She barreled out of the room on a mission to seek and destroy, having not so much as looked in Steph's direction. Steph could hear her mother calling out to nurses in the hallway, eager to unleash her indignant rage.

Rich leaned over his son, inspecting the damage. He let his hardened hand rest on Josh's chest. He gently rubbed it back and forth.

"This used to always calm him down if he had a bad dream. He'd come into our room at night, crying about whatever nightmare he was having. And we'd have him crawl between us and I'd pat his chest like this, and he'd fall right to sleep."

Rich snapped back, the soldier inside pulling up his bootstraps. His spine straightened as he forced a smile, which he offered to Steph. He opened his arms, demanding an embrace. He enveloped her in a tight hug.

"It's going to be okay," he said. "Everything is going to be okay."

"You don't know that, Dad." Steph immediately felt that her comment was too harsh. It should have existed internally. "But let's hope so."

She felt his quavering back muscles attempting to suppress a fit. He retreated from the hug, hiding his sallow expression as if he were succeeding at disguising his tears. Ever since this new trend of emotion began, he always thought he was clever enough to hide it.

"I spotted some vending machines on the way in," said Rich. "I'm gonna grab myself a pop. Be right back."

He rushed out of the room, a yelp echoing as soon as he disappeared. From the hall, Steph could hear her mother's barked orders and her father's bubbling cries as other hospital patrons, visitors, and employees rushed back and forth.

Josh had arrived, and then Steph. People had come, and now people had gone. Steph was alone with Josh, standing in a room she hated, her brother lying in a bed. She stood in deep cogitation, considering the scales of optimism and pessimism, wondering which way they were tipping. She and her brother often sat on opposite sides. Her brother was a programmer, specializing in the development of gaming. The perennial lost boy who refused to grow up. Whereas Steph was proudly logical, both feet planted in reality. Having worked for Loyola-Marymount University as a Senior Budget Analyst, she had a practical career that demanded practical decision making. She made more money than him, which she relished in reminding him of.

But her cynicism felt misplaced without her adversary present to combat it. Perhaps this would persuade her to take a more even position. However, as logical as she could be, she failed at her evaluation of the current odds. Should she be optimistic or pessimistic? Maybe if she stood very still and replayed each moment and the surrounding images: Josh's bleak appearance, Dr. Kaspin's confident plan, her mother's stabbing line of dubious questioning, and her father's vulnerability, maybe she could discover a clue as to which direction the scales were tipping. But as she replayed the tape in her head, she found the outcome to be nebulous every time.

Too early to call, she thought.

She approached her sleeping brother, patting him on the chest just as her father had done. Her gaze lingered across the wall, finally resting on a lazy watercolor painting of a sailboat floating upon a placid surface. She scoffed, upset with herself for finding the image comforting.

CHAPTER THREE

THE COUPE DEVILLE RUMBLED INTO TOWN, THE STEREO thumping the cassette that came with his first car. The band was a popular hard rock '70s band with operatic harmonies, but Josh couldn't remember their name. But he remembered playing the tape, front to back until it had worn out. He was overjoyed to find the cassette tape resting inside the deck, waiting to serenade him as he flew into town. The pulsating bass and grinding guitar wafted through the immense speakers with inspiring, blood-pumping power. He nodded his head with a curled lip, feeling the thump in his chest.

Josh was in awe of the city because it was not a pure metropolis. What he found was equal parts industrial city, urban sprawl, small town, as well as a smattering of any and all significant buildings he had either encountered or seen in famous photographs. It was a melange of memory and nostalgic interest.

An astonished grin crept across Josh's face as he drove by a slew of recognizable buildings: the candy store in downtown San Diego that he used to visit just to ogle, the artisan candle shop that his mother used to venture to after church (he loved watching them dip the wicks into the vats of wax, building size, and eventually carve them with hot scalding hot blades, forming intricate designs that showcased the many colors within), the thrift store in Evanston where he used to spend his lawnmower money on peculiar second-hand items (he always felt like a king because his money seemed to go so far there. This is the store where he purchased a unicycle; he couldn't ride it and failed miserably when he tried, but it made for an interesting conversation piece in the corner of his room).

There were also well-known monuments such as the Chicago Water Tower that he used to bike by on his way to work, the Lincoln Memorial which he visited on his seventh-grade trip to Washington, DC. Fictional buildings also stood throughout town: the enormous newspaper building where his favorite superhero's alter ego worked, the old New York firehouse where his favorite paranormal-fighting-team operated, along with that gigantic tower from that 80's action movie where the terrorists seized control but found that they were in for the ass-kicking of a lifetime when they accidentally crossed paths with a loose-cannon cop who was hiding somewhere inside.

The streets brimmed with buzzing citizens, all of whom wore friendly faces as they rushed off to their respective jobs. They stopped to turn in unison as the Coupe Deville passed by. Every citizen waved to Josh with an over-choreographed welcome. Josh, startled by the immensity of the designed gesture, almost lost control of the Coupe. He blushed as he waved back.

"Hey. Everyone."

The throng nodded in gratitude and went about their day.

It was a balmy, fall day. Deciduous trees lined the street with colors of pleasing ochre, their leaves decorating the streets and sidewalks. The burnt brown and orange, similar to Josh's shag carpet, fomented a feeling of warmth. The slight breeze carried with it a smell of cinnamon, nutmeg, and wet foliage. It smelled like the day of Halloween, Josh's favorite holiday, which he loved because it was a day filled with simmering alacrity and anticipation. As Josh glanced beyond the building and towards the horizon, he could see the twinkling bay of San Diego with her smattering of naval ships. But as he squinted, he also saw the Golden Gate Bridge, which sat next to the Statue of Liberty.

He arrived at his most beloved building of all-time: the Sears Tower. He had once visited the building on an eighth-grade field trip. He had always been so impressed by its looming mass of stygian glass, the hulking frame of American ingenuity, and influential people who worked within. They had since changed the name, but to Josh, it would always be the Sears Tower. It was his dream to work there one day.

A space was open in front of the building. "Rock star parking," he knew his father had always called it. The Coupe Deville drifted into the parking space. Josh stared up at the sky, the tower's glass reflecting darkness, its pointed frame jutting into the sky, pricking the impenetrable blue of the atmosphere as if it meant to rupture the dome under which he was now residing.

"Hey, Joshy," said a familiar voice.

Josh turned to look and took in its source: standing on the curb was a chubby, thirteen-year-old boy with ruddy cheeks, a faded baseball-t, grungy blue jeans, and mischievous eyes. Josh recognized him immediately.

"Andy? Andy Scalco?"

"How goes it, Joshy boy?"

"It can't be you."

Andy had been Josh's best friend in Oregon. Josh had moved there when he was nine and lived in a small town on the coast, until being forced to move to Evanston at the age of thirteen. He remembered that he had moved around a lot, but for the life of him, he couldn't remember why.

But here was Andy, looking exactly the same, even wearing the same clothes that he was the last time Josh saw him.

"In the flesh, Joshy!" Andy exclaimed as he offered his dirty hand.

Josh lit up as he remembered they had a handshake. He engaged, doubtful at first, but what followed was pure magic: two slaps, clasp and spin, snap of the fingers, then a pound with a key-turn and the finishing flourish with the sound effect of an old Model-T.

"aaaOOOOOgggaaaa!" they said in unison.

They burst out laughing. Josh cartoonishly rubbed his eyes in disbelief. Andy had always been the class clown, but this was indeed no joke.

"But wait," said Josh, straining to remember. "Something happened to you. Something terrible." Josh's cogent mind managed to clear the fog. As the answer dawned upon him, his face turned doleful, as if a deep shadow had cascaded over his visage. "There was a fire."

Josh remembered. He had moved that summer to Evanston. Andy was worried that they'd lose touch; Josh would find new friends and forget about him. But Josh had promised Andy they'd stay in touch. He vowed to call Andy every day after school and tell him about his new teachers and friends, while Andy would keep him abreast of all of their old friend's goings-on. They had discussed that perhaps for spring break, Josh could fly back and stay with Andy for the week. But they never got the chance. It was close to Christmas when tragedy struck. Josh remembered that it was around Christmas because he recalled talking to Andy the night before the dreaded incident and the topic had been, "What do you think your parents are getting you for Christmas?"

It was the next day that Josh's phone rang and it wasn't Andy. It was another friend. And he told Josh that there had been a fire at Andy's house. Apparently, a holiday candle was left burning the previous night, and it set fire to a wreath. The home's smoke detectors failed to work and the family, Andy included, suffocated in their sleep. The home, the one that Josh had spent many a sleepover at, with the basement that he and his best friend would try to see how late they could stay up, the one with the large staircase they used to flip slinkies down, had been engulfed in flames.

The friend told Josh that the town was utterly devastated and that the boy and his mom went to the super market to find that they had completely sold out of smoke detectors. He told Josh that even after the house had been burnt to smoldering ash, neighbors still milled about in their robes and pajamas, confused by the senseless tragedy. Josh had only experienced death one other time, when he was eleven-years-old, his grandfather died of cancer. It landed very hard with him, but that was an expected death. Andy was so young, it was incomprehensible.

"I'm a-okay, buddy," said Andy, dusting himself off. "Not a scratch on me."

Josh stood, stunned. Andy swept his red hair back with his grubby hand, flashing a smile that made his freckles bounce.

"You ready for work, dude?" asked Andy.

"Work... right," said Josh, having no idea what he was talking about, but trying to play it off as if he did. He was still reeling, trying to get back up to speed. "Yes, work. Right, let's go. Work time!"

"You alright?" Andy asked with a smile.

"Yep! All good here, my old friend. Quick question: I seem to be a little turned around today, must not have slept well, but where is work?"

"In there," Andy chuckled as he pointed to the top floor of the Sears Tower. "Come on, Joshy, you know that."

"Right! Of course, I do. Work is on the top floor of the Sears Tower. Sounds about right!"

THEY ENTERED A BEDIZENED lobby that was filled with gold and marble. It was beautifully tacky, like the opulent chambers of a tyrant from the Middle East, or a Trumpian hotel. Elevator doors of gold opened, welcoming Josh and Andy. As they entered, Josh admired the beautiful jewel buttons and watched as Andy pushed the button for the top floor. They rocketed skyward, smoothly and quickly.

The doors opened to reveal a standard office setting, only it was humming with saturated life. The floor was sprawling with cubicles, people with familiar faces popping in and out of them like friendly meerkats. Phones rang, and people answered with smiles on their faces. It exuded the feeling of a casual Friday, but where everyone was buying in.

"You alright, Joshy?" asked Andy. "You seem a little dazed, dude."

"This is work?"

"Yeah, man. Come on, let's get you to your cubicle."

As Andy ushered Josh through the aisles of desks and office workers, Josh got a closer look at the people he knew so well. He passed Greg Banks, his jovial camp counselor from when he and Andy went to camp in sixth grade. Greg was in the middle of a story, just about to drop the punchline, but stopped short when he eyed Josh.

"Joshua Husk, Bunk Nine!" he boomed with excitement. "Just did a spontaneous inspection. Clean as a whistle! But I'm afraid you had to pay the 'candy tax.'"

Greg and Josh shared a mischievous, knowing laugh. Josh had always been a messy kid, and when it came to bunk inspection, he always paid Greg off with candy that he smuggled in. As they high-fived, Josh met the gaze of Tyler Willard, his friend from marching band. Tyler played trumpet with Josh, except he was phenomenal whereas Josh had been less than average.

"Well, if it isn't Mr. Third Chair himself," said Tyler with a laugh.

"I'm comin' for that First Chair, Tyler. Better watch your back."

"Well, you'll always be First Chair in my book, bro!"

Another high-five. Josh's head was swimming with rampant stimuli. As he looked around the office, he realized that he recognized every single person. And they ranged in importance, or relevance, in his life. Some of his co-workers weren't even friends of his as much as they were people that gave him a good feeling inside. There was Leia Foth, who had dated a friend of his for a brief time. He always thought she was funny. There was Brandon Bass who was a few grades older than him, but who was a tremendous athlete. He broke varsity football records in Evanston every year that he played and had a way of eschewing the label of cliche-douche-bag-jock. He was charming to Josh in the hallways, saying, "Sup, man," when he saw him. Then there were people he didn't know personally but who represented a cozy feeling to Josh.

In a neighboring cubicle sat Pat Perlola, the game show

host from Josh's favorite game show, *London Bridges Falling Down*. It was a game show where guests had a limited amount of time to answer questions, and the more questions you answered incorrectly, the quicker the styrofoam bridges crumbled. It was an odd show that was obviously underfunded and outdated, but Josh loved to watch when he was home sick from school. There was Lou Featherman, the news anchor from San Diego. He had slicked-back, silver hair, which sat atop a massive forehead. Whenever the news came on, Josh knew it was time for bed; this gave him a warm feeling as he could hear Lou Featherman recounting the day's events from his bed as he drifted off to sleep. And finally, next to Lou, was the famous Chef from Josh's favorite brand of canned pasta. He wore his signature white hat and chef's outfit with an overly-curled mustache. When he saw Josh, he brought his fingers to his mouth and kissed them with a stereotypical, Italian flourish.

But the best was yet to come as from around the corner appeared Big Boy Bear.

"Josh!" exclaimed the elephantine, stuffed bear.

Big Boy Bear was a stuffed animal that was bought for him when he was six-years-old and had come down with a terrible cold. When he got better, he remembered someone saying, "You see? He healed you! He made you be a big boy!" So Josh christened him "Big Boy Bear." He took the bear everywhere, often being lost and then found, or dropped and dirtied. Years of being heavily involved in the day-to-day of young Josh's life had led to rips, holes, and stains in Big Boy's hide. But now, here he was, a massive bear lumbering through a traditional office setting, looking as good as new.

"Big Boy?"

"In the flesh. Or the stuffing, I suppose!"

The entire office stopped to laugh with Josh.

"So, how are you today, my friend?" asked Big Boy Bear.

"Can't complain. Just... another normal day at the office, I guess."

"Tell me about it," said Big Boy. "You wouldn't happen to have the time, would ya, Josh?"

"I sure don't, but let me tell ya if I had a watch it would be set to 'Coffee O'clock,'" quipped Josh.

Booming laughter filled the office as if everyone had been tuned in and heard Josh's terrible joke. Josh was startled by the reaction. Never had he received such a unanimously positive response to his humor. Everyone in the office had buckled over to Josh's corny one-liner. As the laughter subsided, they looked to Josh, who lit up, sensing their want for more.

"I mean, don't even talk to me until I've had my coffee. Talking to me without coffee is like talking to a zombie," said Josh. He then acted like a zombie, trudging through the office. "Braaaiiinnnsss. Cafffeeeiinnnnneeee. Aaannnnddd bbbr-rraaiiiinnnssss."

Again, sonorous laughter. His coworkers voraciously lapped it up, consumed by Josh's unheralded humor. The entire office crept closer as if Josh were a bonfire in the cold wilderness; they absorbed his warmth. He possessed a gravitational pull, bringing them in ever-so firmly. Josh held court like a veteran comic.

"Now I'm afraid that coffee isn't enough. Pretty soon I'm going to have to switch to gasoline," he joked, getting a laugh. He then acted as if he were in line at a Starbucks, simulating a customer exchange. "'Excuse me, barista, I'll have a small cheese Danish and a Venti Unleaded Roast!'"

This was a killer. People fell to their knees, unable to physically deal with Josh's hilarity. Their faces flooded with crimson red, their sucking lips gasping for air. Josh was aston-ished by the destructive impact that his jokes had made.

"That's enough!" boomed a voice.

Josh looked up to see Mr. Weeks, his fifth-grade P.E. teacher.

"I guess I must have missed the memo that we were going to spend the day pullin' each other's puds!" yelled Mr. Weeks.

Mr. Weeks had always been no-nonsense. He was an infamous stickler for kids who were a distraction, as Josh often was.

Andy nudged Josh, flashing a grin. "Looks like Weeks has something lodged up his butt."

"What else is new?" Josh snickered. But he stopped as he felt Mr. Weeks's gaze fall upon him.

"This is why sales are so low," said Mr. Weeks. "This horsin' around, grab ass, bullshit is why we're not living up to our potential. Let's go, in the conference room. Hustle it up! That means you, Husk. You too, Scalco." Josh threw Andy a familiar face of "Oh shit, I think we're in trouble."

"He's such a blowhard," said Andy with a shrug and a roll of the eyes.

"I know, but I don't wanna get in trouble. Maybe we shouldn't sit together when we get in there."

"Bullshit," said Andy. "We can't let old man Weeks win. You know he just likes to yell. He ain't gonna do shit."

Office workers quickly shuffled into the conference room. Big Boy Bear took a seat in the corner next to Josh and Andy, along the back wall. In the middle of the room rested a large, dark, walnut table. A wall of windows looked out onto the hodgepodge city. The room was filled, but eerily quiet, everyone staring at their hands as Mr. Weeks paced back-

and-forth. His eyes burned with menace as he stared the office down.

"We've been slacking," he said. "Sales have been way, way down. I look around, and all I see are people half-assing everything. I'm tired, sick and tired, of all the pud pullin'! I see people giving minimum effort. Pat Perlola, where are you?"

The game show host raised his hand, flashing his classic afternoon-television-smile.

"Pat, you wipe that shit-eating grin off your face. You've been doggin' it on the phones. I need you to get your act together. Do you know the bind that we're in, people?!"

Mr. Weeks moved to the whiteboard at the front of the room and reached for a hanging pull-cord. He unrolled a large canvas chart that stretched across the wall. The chart had no data on it, merely a large, red arrow that trended harshly downward.

"We're riding a sinking ship, people!" screamed Mr. Weeks. "We need to get our act together! Big Boy Bear..."

Big Boy's head raised and winced, waiting for the strike.

"Big Boy, you've been sucking ass. Where's the hustle? You're supposed to be the glue of this office? Well, I don't see it. I don't see a Big Boy Bear. All I see is a big fat pain in my ass!"

Big Boy Bear lowered his head in shame.

The room was silent as Mr. Weeks softened. He looked to be giving up.

"Look, I know I could stand up here all day and scream myself hoarse. I could go one-by-one, call you guys all sorts of names, but you and I both know that it won't make a lick of difference. So, I'm just gonna ask... and this will be the only time I ever do this, but... does anyone want to take a crack at this?"

The room was confused, caught off-guard.

"I mean it," Mr. Weeks assured everyone. "If anyone thinks they can somehow inspire this group, by all means, give it a shot. Because I'm out of answers here, people. So? Does anyone want to give this a chance?"

Andy nudged Josh. "Do it," whispered Andy.

"What? No. Are you kidding?"

"Come on. Pussy."

"That's ridiculous. What would I even say?"

"Do it," said Andy, nudging him harder in the ribs.

"Ow!"

This caught the attention of Mr. Weeks. "Hey, cut the grab-ass back there, Husk!"

"Sorry," muttered Josh, sinking in his chair.

"And sit up straight," said Mr. Weeks. "Matter of fact, stand up, Husk. Get the hell up here. You always seem to have something funny to say, so how about you say it to the group? Let's go, mister. Hop to it!"

Josh slowly rose to his feet, heaving a petulant sigh. He threw Andy a look.

"What the fuck, dude?" he whispered.

"Got ya," said Andy with a wink.

Josh slinked to the front of the room, taking his time. "Move it, Husk," said Mr. Weeks. "We ain't got all day!"

Josh reached the front of the room, turning to look into vacant eyes. There were no answers out in this sea of gaping faces. He cleared his throat and began to form words with his lips, but no sound came out. His heart pounded in his chest. He turned to inspect the chart, but there were just as little answers there as there were in the crowd of blank, familiar faces.

"Um. So like," Josh stammered as he began. "Work... we all hate it, but we gotta do it, ya know?"

"Mmhmm," someone hummed with agreement in the room.

Josh looked to Andy who stifled his laughter in the back of the room. Mr. Weeks stared daggers, the embers of rage beginning to ignite. But at least the coworkers were listening, nodding their heads. He had their attention.

"Look," he said. "We all have a job to do. And that job is... what?"

Silence clung to the room as they expected Josh to answer his own question. But Josh was sincerely asking.

"Someone say what it is," he said. "The job we do. Someone say it."

"Sales," said Pat Perlola, the game show host.

"Okay, sure. But what else?"

"Customer service," said Leia, his friend's old girlfriend.

"Right. Yes. But I mean, what is it exactly that we do here?"

Ponderous, ruminating thought ensued as the office considered his philosophical question.

"We sell," said Lou Featherman, the news anchor, proudly.

"Okay, but what do we sell?"

"Ourselves," said Brandon Bass, the nice upper-classman.

"Aha," someone said from somewhere in the room. Now there was intense nodding.

"Sure, but that's not what I mean. Here's what I'm asking: what is it that we do in this building? Why are we here? Why are we even in this room right now? What... are we doing?"

Involved, emphatic nodding infected his coworkers as they took what they thought he was saying to heart.

"Wow," said Leia. "Okay, now I think I know where you're going with this."

"Yes-a," said the Italian Chef who made microwavable food and was now beginning to cry. "It's-a like-a, why are we-a here-a?! What are we-a doing with-a our lives-a?!"

"I guess, I've never really thought about it like that," said Pat Perlola, visibly drawing into himself.

There was a hum amongst the room as everyone comforted one another in their linked, existential questioning. People began to cry as they hugged, some fully embracing and passionately kissing, the preciousness and fragility of existence now apparent to them.

"Josh is right!" said Big Boy Bear. "We have to live for today. Because that's all we are promised."

A hand landed on Josh's shoulder. It was Mr. Weeks, who had shed a tear.

"Powerful stuff there, Husk. And as provocative as it is, maybe that silver tongue can inspire us to get some work done? It can't all be bad, right? How's about a little something to get us motivated and back out there? Something to get us going? Whaddaya say there, Josh?"

"Yeah, Joshy," called Andy, ironically smiling from the back of the room. "Any other nuggets of wisdom?"

Josh reeled, wracking his brain for any modicum of a motivational speech. He surveyed the group of tearful coworkers, all leaning forward, eager for his next philosophical bombshell.

"I guess I do have something," said Josh, straining to remember. In truth, he had found something. But the denizen fog had returned and was preventing him from fleshing out the origin of the memory he had stumbled upon. "I don't remember where I heard this, but someone once told it to me... Maybe it was some famous guy, I don't know. But..." He trailed off, turning to look at the chart. He inspected it, again arriving at his inner conclusion. "Apparently you, or I mean we, failed. But that's only natural. It's the nature of the game."

"The game?" asked Lou Featherman.

"Uh, yeah, the game of business," Josh stammered. It was loose footing, but somewhere lodged in his brain was this speech. He knew it to be his only reliable escape route. "It's a game based on failure. Ya know, .300 hitters get into the hall of fame. And that means that they've managed to fail seventy percent of the time. The difference between those players and the players who we forget about is that those players, the .300 hitters, know how to come back from failure. They know how to refocus and adjust for their next at-bat."

Emphatic nodding rippled through the room like a dashboard of bobble-heads.

"I don't know what it is we do here, but I don't want this failure to shape us. I want it to make us even better. Greater."

"Yes-a! He's a-right!" said the Italian Chef.

"Next time we step up to the plate, we need to keep our heads down. Our eyes need to be on the ball. And we can't drop our back shoulder."

"You're damn right!" said Brandon Bass.

"And that applies to other sports! And jobs! And life! If you fall down, you don't just lie there! You get the heck back up!"

Hoots and hollers reverberated throughout the conference room. His coworkers were now frothing at the mouth. Josh paced like a megalomaniacal preacher of a super church. He soaked in their radiant love, now fueling his feverish performance.

"Now look here," he said, embracing the raucous crowd. "I love you crazy bunch'a SOB's, and I'd do anything for ya. So let's get out there, do whatever it is that we do, and give 'em hell! Whaddaya say?!"

A champagne bottle popped from out of nowhere. Then, several others. Corks flew, and bubbly spilled. The coworkers rushed to Josh, dousing him with champagne as if he had just pitched a no-hitter in the World Series. Everyone clung to each other, bouncing and shaking, an outpour of booze and love. Andy managed to squeeze through the madness and find Josh.

"Rousing speech, Joshy!"

"Thanks, dude! I don't know where I heard it, but I swear-"

Mr. Weeks slipped through the jostling and enveloped Josh and Andy in a tight hug.

"I always knew you had it in you, kid! The both of you. Well done! Hey, I tell you what, you and Andy take the day off. You've done enough here."

"Really? Are you sure?"

But Mr. Weeks had not heard Josh's reply, having poured champagne down his throat and across his face. He joined the chaos, celebrating with the rest of the office.

"You hear that?" asked Andy. "We get the day off!"

They cued up their secret handshake as salutary punctuation to victory.

"What should we do?" asked Josh.

"Come on, Joshy, let's hit the town."

Josh grinned as he surveyed the excitement. Never had he created such jubilant hysteria. He savored the celebration as flecks of champagne kissed his face.

CHAPTER FOUR

FROTHY SODA SPILLED ONTO JOSH'S SLEEPING FACE. THE foam hissed from the bottle of Coca-Cola held above his head by his bumbling father.

"Rich, what the hell are you doing?!" yelled Lisa.

Rich scrambled to reverse the situation. His elbows tensed, clasping to a bottle of volcanic Coke, fizzing onto his unconscious son's face, the bottle spilling its bubbling contents from the creases of the cap, his hand cupped in an attempt to catch the falling remnants.

"I'm sorry," mumbled Rich as he tried to correct his mistake, tightening the cap and loosening it again. "The damn machine dropped it too hard or something. I don't know, it just exploded."

"He has soda all over his face, Rich."

"I see that, Lisa! I'm not blind, dammit."

Rich tried to correct the misstep by wiping Josh's face with a stuffed animal that had been resting by his son's side.

"Rich, no!" yelled Lisa. "That's his Big Boy Bear."

Lisa reproachfully snatched the stuffed animal from his

hands. She pulled a batch of soft tissues from the bedside table and gently dabbed at her son's face with sedulous affection, simultaneously shooing Rich away like a diseased pigeon.

"Oh come on, look at that thing," said Rich, motioning to the bear. "It looks like a leper. I'm sure it can take a little pop."

Rich was correct in that Big Boy Bear looked worse for wear. His bear was ratty and rugged, his light brown fluff matted down to a bleak grey. Stuffing bled from the stitching that had split, looking as if the bear had been a member of Sonny Corleone's ill-fated crew. An eye had gone missing, and the button nose was crooked and chipped.

"I'm just saying, it's a depressing enough site already. He doesn't need a dead teddy bear lying next to him."

"He would want it," said Lisa as she gingerly tucked the bear into the pit of his arm. The presence of the bear also gave her comfort. He would always be here, watching over him.

"I'm sorry, Lisa. Jesus."

She threw him a reproachful glare of severe warning. Rich stumbled and stammered.

"I mean, jeez. Jeez, Lisa."

Rich thrust his hands into his pockets and meandered to the middle of the room. He looked to Steph to share a look of exasperation, but she was sitting by the window, staring at the parking lot, lost in thought.

"I didn't mean to take the guy's name in vain, Lees, but I've never heard him complain," said Rich, offering it up as a half-baked joke. He looked to Steph, fishing for a reaction, but she didn't seem to be listening.

"That 'guy' is our lord and savior," said Lisa with bristling rancor. "And perhaps now isn't the best time to joke about Him."

Rich nodded, accepting the blow. A predicated knockout of his prescient suspicions that he was not wanted and maybe it would be for the best if he retreated and kept to himself. He drifted over to the television, turning it on and fiddling with the channels. It was an older set; the turning, dial knob clicked as it shifted, jumping rigidly from channel to channel, most of which came in shrouded in fuzz.

"What are you doing, Dad?" asked Steph.

"There's a game on. I need something to take my mind off this stuff. Besides, I read that noise can make them come out of their coma."

"Where did you read that?" asked Lisa.

"The internet. I was googling stuff about comas. There were a ton of articles about it."

He found a baseball game; the Cubs were playing. He increased the volume until the speakers were blaring and buzzing.

"Rich, turn it down."

"What if it helps?"

"It's not."

"Yeah, it's too loud, Dad."

"Besides, he doesn't like baseball," said Lisa.

Rich recoiled. "He loves baseball, Lisa."

"No. He doesn't. He played baseball when he was a kid, but he doesn't love it. When was the last time you saw him watch a baseball game?"

"The last time we went. A couple years ago."

"I'll rephrase: when was the last time you saw him watch baseball on television?"

Rich thought, then grew truculent, blushing with anger. He turned his back to her, defiantly raising the volume.

"Dad!"

"Rich!"

"Fine!"

He muted the set, slinking to the corner with querulous posturing. His tan arms folded against his chest, leaning against the alabaster walls. He looked to Lisa who gave him a slow shake of disappointment. She then turned to Steph, disturbed by her daughter's deflated demeanor. Rich had unleashed a cloud of acrimony upon the room, blanketing them with a toxic pall. Much like their parental dynamic, it was up to her to fix everything.

"How's work, hun?" she asked Steph. "Hun" was reserved for endearing moments. Whenever deployed, Steph knew her mother was really trying.

"Fine," she said. "The university has had me at supervisor for eight months now, and we've already slashed the budget by nearly twenty-five percent."

"Twenty-five? That's a lot," said Lisa.

"Yeah. Basically, it was my idea to get rid of the Film School. So once we did that, we had a lot more room to divert to other programs."

"You got rid of the Film School? Isn't that their big thing?" asked Rich.

"No, that's Columbia and DePaul," said Steph, flatly. "School of Business, Communications, Liberal Arts, are Loyola's primary programs. We also have a great Law School."

"Isn't Liberal Arts the same kinda thing? It's acting, right?" asked Rich.

"It can be. It's dance, music, theater."

"Yeah, remember, Rich? Mary Graham's boy was a Liberal Arts major."

"Wait, which kid was that? Was he the one who came out as gay but then married a woman?"

"No, that was the older boy, Paul," said Lisa. "Stephen became a teacher. He was in that nasty car accident where he lost his big toe. He saw us at the grocery store, and he has that weird walk now."

"Oh, right. So, the university is doing away with Liberal Arts, huh?"

"Film School. They're getting rid of the Film School because it was hemorrhaging money."

"Well, that stinks for those kids," said Rich.

"There are plenty of places in Chicago for them to continue their education. They knew the risks of going to a new program."

"Do they have you working from home?" asked Lisa.

"No, although they've said that's an option."

"Oh, so you're working in the city..." said Lisa, feigning surprise.

"Yes. Why do you say it like that, mother?"

"Well, that's just surprising to me because you say you can't swing by after work anymore. That's all."

"That's because they moved me to the south side campus, Mom. I used to swing by when I worked north side. I can't do that anymore."

"You can't or you won't? That's only an extra twenty minutes? That's too long of a drive to see us?" she asked.

"Wait... There are two campuses? Is that common?" asked Rich.

"It's more than twenty minutes. Since we moved to Bolingbrook, that would mean I'd get off at five, drive to you, which takes thirty to forty minutes."

"That's not true," said Lisa. "Rich, how long does it take to drive that?"

"Twenty-five? Maybe thirty? I don't know. Haven't done it in years. I have no need to go to the south side. I used to know a dentist down on there, but that was years ago. Lisa, what was his name? It was something funny... Dr. Booth! That's right. It always made me laugh because it rhymed with tooth."

"Okay, let's say thirty," said Steph. "So I see you guys for probably a half an hour because then I need to sit in traffic for an hour and forty-five minutes to get home in time to make dinner for Levi. That sounds logical and like a lot of fun for me, Mom."

"All I'm saying is that you could make more of an effort to see us. Why did you stop coming to Sunday dinners? Josh always manages to make it, why can't you?"

"Because Shawn's sister comes over Sunday night and we watch a movie. It's our own little tradition. Why don't you come and see us, Mom? We have the spare room, we'd love to have you."

"I don't think that's fair. We're not the ones who decided to move all the way to Bolingbrook."

Steph turned taciturn, staring back out the window. She knew her mother hated that move to the suburbs and saw it as an aggressive gesture to separate herself further from the family. This wasn't entirely unfounded.

"So, is Shawn watching Levi?" asked Lisa.

"Yeah."

"Are you getting a divorce?" asked Lisa.

"Jesus, Lisa," sighed Rich.

"I'll ask you to please not do that again, Rich. Don't make me send you home."

By turning the attention back on Rich and his abhorrent blasphemy, Lisa felt she had spared herself from pushing. Rich shook his head as he brought his attention back to the

muted baseball game. Much like the doctors she often deni-
grated, Lisa was not gifted in conversation.

"You know," said Lisa, carefully beginning to pry.
"There's counseling through the church. Whatever it is that
you two are going through, it's not worth putting poor Levi
through. You have to think of the grand scheme of things."

Steph scowled at this. Her mother was an inveterate
patronizer, using her piousness to imperiously criticize. She
had used it liberally on her daughter ever since Steph
decided not to attend DePaul University, a Catholic college.
Then, when given the opportunity to work for Loyola or
DePaul, sensing her mother's excitement to both work for a
Catholic school and work closer to home, she deferred to the
school with the prominent south side campus, although,
much to her chagrin she was staffed at the north side office,
which was even closer to her parent's Evanston home.

"Mom, I really don't want to get into this right now. And
with you of all people. You're not exactly the ideal audience."

"What is that supposed to mean?"

"Let's take it easy," said Rich, sensing the tension, but
also having a sideways smile that said he was enjoying Lisa
getting herself into a bit of trouble.

"Never mind," said Steph, retreating her gaze back to the
window.

"No, please. Tell me. I'd like to know why I'm not the
ideal audience for your marital problems. Is it because I'm
your mother?" she genuinely asked. "You don't think I can
understand?"

"Mom, it should be pretty obvious. I really just don't
want to talk about it right now."

"But you already said it, so now you have to defend it.
Why am I not the ideal audience?"

"Because you guys haven't had, like, the greatest situation. And if all your advice is going to be is 'just grin and bear it,' or, "turn to the church," I'm not really interested."

Lisa's eyes narrowed. "We don't all get to be with our soulmate," she said.

"I second that," said Rich as he fiddled with the television set. Lisa rolled her eyes, shaking her head as she turned to Josh. He was such a peacemaker. He would tell a joke or change the subject if he were awake. He was so gifted in social settings, she always admired that about him. She was never like that as a girl. She touched the gold cross hanging from her neck. She often did it as a silent prayer for resolve. She closed her eyes and quickly regrouped, conjuring his peacemaking abilities.

"Maybe Shawn should bring Levi by," she said, mustering a gentle smile.

"No, I don't want him seeing his uncle like this. He loves Josh."

"I just don't understand, Stephanie," said Lisa, carefully this time. "What happened? What did he do? Or was it something you did? Were you unfaithful? It happens sometimes."

"Does it?" asked Rich, suddenly bewildered.

"Well... to people. It happened to the Barkley's. Our group said a prayer for them and they managed to come back from it. I'm just saying, Steph if that's the problem then maybe seeking forgiveness on a larger scale might allow you to look inward and find the problem."

Steph had been poked one too many times. Her hackle went up.

"He's self-absorbed."

"Shawn? Shawn is self-absorbed?" asked Lisa.

"So," said Rich, staring at the television, now landing on the daytime game show, *London Bridges Falling Down*.

"I thought he was having an affair," said Steph.

"You 'thought?'" Lisa asked.

"Yes. He was always texting someone, and when I'd ask who he was texting, he wouldn't say. Or he'd just say 'it's someone from work.' And so when he was in the shower, I checked his texts, and I found out who it was."

"Was he?" asked Rich. "Cheating?"

Steph sighed, really not wanting to go further into this.

"Yes. Well, no, but kinda."

Lisa and Rich shared a look of confusion. Rich threw up his hands as if to say, "What the fuck does that mean?" Steph witnessed the exchange, which was oddly comforting, seeing them on the same side.

"He was emotionally cheating on me," she said, predicting the raised brows of confusion that Lisa would, and did, wear.

"What does that mean?" she asked.

"He was flirting with this woman from work, sending little jokey messages back and forth, pictures and videos and things. And when I confronted him about it, he tried to play it off like it was nothing, but it was evident that he had a thing for her. I told him to stop, but he didn't. We tried to work through it, but every time we talked about it, it turned into a fight. So I told him to go live somewhere else for a bit while we tried to work things out. I don't want Levi around us when we're like that. It was getting a little ugly."

"So that's it," said Lisa. "'Emotional cheating?'"

Steph nodded, waiting for her mother's comment, which finally came.

"Your generation is so ridiculous."

Rich pushed off the wall that he was leaning on, back on his feet. He seized control of the middle of the room, his hands clasped together, ready to motivate.

"Here's the deal, sweetheart," he began. "Marriage is

work. And it can be really tough work, there's no doubt about it. Sometimes it's not fun work. I'll tell ya, there have been some tough years for your mother and me. Lord knows-"

"Rich..." she said warning.

"There have been times that I just wanted to run away," he said, boldly. "Go to someplace far off, just hit a tree-line and take off into the woods, never come back." He laughed, but no one shared in it. They only stared, eagerly waiting for him to arrive at his point.

"I've had those thoughts, is what I'm saying. There were times when things were hard when you guys were kids, and Josh was having trouble in school, and you were throwing a fit, and your mother was... being your mother. I'd be driving home from work, and I'd think, 'What if I kept driving? What if I just blew past my exit and kept driving and never came back? Started a new life. New name. New town. New people.' Men used to do that sort of thing back in the day. Start a new family. I've had those thoughts, Steph. More times than I can count."

"'More times than you can count?'" asked Lisa.

"Well, maybe not that many."

"How many, Rich? How many times did you think of taking off?"

"It's not like that. I wasn't seriously considering it. It was just a thought."

"Give me an estimate."

"It wasn't a ton, Lisa."

"Give me a number."

"It wasn't like I thought about it a million times or something."

"So less than a million. That's great."

"I don't know! A couple hundred?"

"A couple hundred?!"

"I don't know, Lisa! I'm just talking!"

"I'll say," she muttered as she returned to Josh. Rich fumbled, trying to remember his original point.

"What I'm trying to say... I just meant that... if you..."

"What is it you're trying to say, Dad?"

A light bulb went off, he had it. "What I'm trying to say is... well, things change is all."

"Uh huh. And what if things change for the worse?" asked Steph.

"Well, then you... well, you change with them. Or, you just... you don't run away, is all. That's it. Look, I'm just talking. I just want to help here, people."

"Nice, Rich," said Lisa with a wry smile.

"Can't a guy just try to help his daughter? Jesus."

"That's it!" Lisa boomed. "Out!"

Rich's shoulders sheepishly slumped. He looked to Steph whose gaze had returned to the window. Lisa leered at him, expectantly, waiting for him to follow orders like a good soldier. Rich sighed and reached for what was left of the Coca-Cola, but not before Lisa snagged it. Not because she wanted it, but because she wanted him to have nothing. There was nothing for him in this room. He shook his head in disbelief and sauntered out of the room, cradling what masculinity he had left.

RICH WALKED the halls of the hospital, crestfallen, wending towards nowhere. He watched as strangers scurried and limped past. Everyone had someplace to be, everyone going as fast as they could go; even if that wasn't very fast at all, they seemed to be doing their best. He noted that the building's inhabitants were harboring their own experience, possessing dissimilar feelings, almost as if they existed on different timelines. It was an environment of sequestered emotion. The patrons and workers were like schools of fish, moving around one another to get to a place of dire significance. Some slow, some fast, but all with intention.

He passed rooms with newborn babies and their new parents. He remembered when he was a new parent. He had been terrified, Lisa clutching his hand as tight as she ever had. When they first gave him Josh, he felt an overwhelming fear that he was going to fuck it up. Not just by dropping the newborn, but that he wouldn't be a worthy father of such a little, adorable being. Josh looked at him, which to Rich felt like a poker player pushing his chips into the middle of the table, all-in, awaiting Rich's move. "Well, what are you gonna do?"

He passed rooms filled with the elderly, their time coming to an end. He remembered the passing of his parents. The finality of their passing. What struck him most about death wasn't the usual worry of "where do you go after you die?" It was the reality of being unable to talk to them. Or hear their voice. They had moved away and were unable to keep in touch. But not because they didn't want to, but because it was impossible. That reality was the most heartbreaking element to Rich. The death of conversation.

And here he was, passing rooms of life and death, all while his son sat somewhere in the middle.

He found the vending machines, perusing them only for a moment before deciding on another Coke. He inserted a dollar and selected a bottle, but the machine refused to release it. Rich realized that it was $1.25. He dropped his head down in supplication to Lisa's god for things to be just a tad bit easier for him.

"Need a quarter?" asked a kind voice behind him.

Rich looked to see a man in his mid-forties. He had wrinkles around his eyes and a bright smile. He was wearing a dirtied baseball uniform, digging through his wallet.

"Because I have some extra change, I think," said the kind man.

"If you have a quarter to spare, that would be much appreciated."

He tossed Rich a shiny quarter, and he inserted it immediately, which brought his soda barreling down the machine.

"Be careful when you open these," said Rich. "This machine has a way of shaking them up pretty good."

"Got ya. Thanks, stranger."

The man inserted his money and looked over his options. Rich started to leave, but couldn't pull himself away from the man. Something demanded that he connect with him.

"So, you expecting a call-up to the big leagues this year?" Rich joked, referencing the full uniform.

Rich's joke took the man by surprise, but then he gave a hearty laugh. "You know it. Put me in coach, I'm ready to play."

They laughed, sportsman camaraderie blossoming between them.

"But seriously, you coming from a softball game or something? Slowpitch?" asked Rich.

"No, no. It's just something the coaches wear. I coach my son's little league team."

Rich lit up, his eyebrows nearly bumping into his non-receding hairline.

"Little league, eh? I used to coach my son's little league team."

"Oh yeah?"

"Absolutely. Some of the best times, I'll tell ya. Loved every minute of it. We took county one year."

"No kidding," said the man, adopting an appeasing tone for the old-timer, but also with growing interest.

"God, what I'd give to do it again," said Rich. "I coached All-Stars two years in a row. I always stressed fundamentals. That was my thing. That's what they need at that age, before high school, you know? That way they understand the game, but also have fun."

"Preach, brother, preach. I've been trying to do the same thing, but all they want to do is swing for the fences."

"What's your boy play?" Rich asked, getting excited and comfortable.

"First base."

"So he's a lefty?"

"Sure is," the man said with a proud smile.

"That's what my boy, Josh, played. He wanted to pitch so bad, but I didn't want him getting hurt or burning out his arm in case he wanted to play high school or college ball."

"I know. If he stays interested, I want him to have that option too. Schools will pay for a lefty, especially one who has a lot of arm left. So if he gets a free education out of the deal..."

They quietly nodded in agreement at the sound sense of the plan.

"First base, oh man..." said Rich, wistfully. Then he quickly turned worrisome. "What brings you in? The boy okay?"

"He'd been having stomach aches," said the man. "We were midway through a game, and he couldn't take it anymore. He asked me to take him to the hospital. I asked, 'Are you sure?' And he said he was. I was surprised by how serious he was. It wasn't like him, you know?"

"So, what happened?"

"Appendicitis."

"Oh, Jesus."

"Yeah, scary stuff."

"So he needs surgery, then?"

"Afraid so. He's going under tomorrow. It's the type of thing that, the doctor says, doesn't go wrong. It's pretty close to a guarantee that it'll be fine. But still... I'm nervous. I just wish I could do it for him, you know? I hate that he has to go through this."

Rich nodded understanding, but also incredibly jealous of the man's innocuous health concerns. How he wished that his worry was over such a minor, benign situation. The man didn't know real uncertainty. He was manufacturing it as a form of self-preservation to steel himself from the surprise of the minuscule possibility of things going wrong. But Rich was experiencing the worst-case scenario. He was living the man's nightmare.

"Does he hit?" asked Rich.

"He does," said the man, thankful for the shift in topic. "He smacks the hell out of the ball."

"Yeah, that was Josh's weakness. Great fielder, really fast, but never could hit all that well. He was always scared of the ball. No matter what sport he played, he always played scared. Football, he ran scared. Basketball, scared of charging in. Soccer, afraid of getting hit in the face with the ball. Baseball, scared of getting hit by the pitch. Being a lefty, the kids always seem to have difficulty locating, so he got hit quite a bit. It happens."

"Yeah, kids are erratic at that age. Especially the ones trying to throw curve balls and whatnot."

"Josh could never hang in there. They'd throw in, and he'd get spooked, then he was an easy strikeout. I'll never forget when he made All-Stars. I was coaching, and I played him at first. He was actually having a pretty good game. He led off the game with a single. I was proud of him, watching him grinning like an idiot on first base. He gave me a thumbs up, enthusiastic but also trying to play it cool. I loved watching him act like the pros we used to watch on TV. Anyways, we're up early, but then our pitcher gives up four runs. But we manage to come back in the eighth. We're down by one run. So in the ninth, we load the bases. We have two outs and who's up, but Josh. I take him aside, and I say, 'You can do this, buddy. Just wait for your pitch. Be aggressive when it comes.' Well, he goes up there, and he watches three strikes come right down the pipe. Doesn't even swing the bat. The moment was too big for him. God how I wished I could have taken that at-bat for him. The poor kid was just distraught. He looked like Charlie Brown as he sulked back to the dugout. He was crying, feeling like he let all of his friends down. It just seemed so unfair."

"What'd you say to him?" asked the man.

"I knew he didn't want to be lectured, so I addressed the team, but of course I was mainly talking to him. I said, 'Look, we failed. Including me. We all failed. But that's only natural. It's the nature of the game. It's a game based on failure. Ya know, .300 hitters get into the hall of fame. And that means they've managed to fail seventy percent of the time. The difference between those players and the players who we forget about is that those players, the .300 hitters, know how to come back from failure. They know how to refocus and adjust for their next at-bat. And I don't want this failure to shape you guys. At least not in a bad way. I want it to make you even better. Greater. So next time we step up to the plate, we need to keep our heads down. Our eyes need to be on the ball. And we can't drop our back shoulder. We need to be aggressive. And that applies to other sports, and it applies to life. If you fall down, you don't just lie there. You get the heck back up.'"

"Hell yeah," said the man. "Did that shake him out of it?"

"Kinda. The boys all gave him a pat on the back, and he was teary on the way home, but we stopped and got some milkshakes. I started telling him jokes and stories about when I played ball, times I'd messed up or made a fool of myself. I had him laughing in no time." Rich grinned at his memory.

"Does it ever get easier?" asked the man. "It feels like even the smallest thing has me freaking out."

"You never stop worrying about your kids," said Rich. "No matter what. Because no matter how old they get, they're still your kids. It's especially hard when they're going through something you can't do anything about."

The fathers stood there in silence.

"And what about your boy? What's he up to now?" the man asked.

"Gaming engineer. Works in video games."

"Oh, I'd imagine that's every boy's dream job."

"Yeah. Unfortunately, he's why we're here today, too."

"What's he in for?" asked the man.

The question Rich had been dreading, but he managed to manipulate his mind into an alternate reality for the time being.

"Broken collarbone. Riding his bike to work, he fell off, hit the ground hard. He's alright though. We should be out in a couple of days."

"Oh, that's great. I envy you."

As easy as that. It felt real in that moment. It felt terrific, actually.

CHAPTER FIVE

ANDY LED JOSH THROUGH THE STREETS OF THE aberrant megacity as if he were a hired tour guide leading him through a meticulously detailed theme park. He pointed out the plethora of options they had before them, attempting to find something that would pique Josh's interest. The day's entertainment choices were boundless. However, Josh was still struggling to take it all in and make cognitive sense of it. He followed Andy around the smooth sidewalks, gawking at the buildings that held various notoriety in his memory, many of them looming in his brain with great immensity, and others that housed only the slightest bit of significance. Everywhere Josh turned, his jaw was agape at the scrupulous detail of this new, sprawling universe.

"Check it out," said Andy. "The old library!"

There it was with its recognizable, antiquated structure: four massive columns that made it look as if it had been ripped from the center of Ancient Rome. Josh had always loved going to the library, but this one especially. They had a computer lab with countless games, walls of movies to check out at your leisure, as well as a large stand of comic books. Sometimes he'd get dropped off in the summer, the building serving as a makeshift babysitter. Many children spent their summers at the community pool, while Josh spent his June through August bathing in the silence of graphic novels and heroes in underwear.

"Wanna go inside?" asked Andy. "We could play some Oregon Trail. Just like old times."

"Nah. We kinda figured it out, didn't we? All you gotta do is hunt and fish a ton, and you make it to the coast just fine."

"Okay. Well, how about we swing by the old Gas N' Go?"

On the corner sat the Gas N' Go, a gas station that had the best candy aisle anyone had ever seen. Josh and Andy chuckled as they ran up to the front window to peer inside. It was just as he remembered. Not only that, but the aisles were teeming with all of the limited-time-only candy that Josh had almost forgotten. They even had his favorite peanut butter candy. They were the ones that came out as a promotional tie-in for an action movie in the early '90s, the one about the big muscly guy who was sent from the future to terminate an unborn child. They only lasted for a couple months. They were balls of peanut butter, covered in chocolate, with a piece of pretzel in the middle. He used to buy three bags at a time. Unbelievable.

"What do you say, Joshy? My treat."

"I'm not really hungry."

"Well, we could catch a movie."

Across the street sat the old State Theater. It had closed down since Josh moved from San Diego. But here it was, standing its ground, open for business, and displaying the titles of his top five favorite films.

"No, it's okay. I'd rather just walk around, get some fresh air. I don't think I'm feeling too great."

Andy nodded as they strolled through the streets. Josh felt encroaching nausea for reasons he could not define. None of this was making any sense. While the buildings and familiar faces fomented feelings of warmth and comfort, he could not help but feel exhausted by the amount of familiarity and its impetuous stitching. The lurid colors of the buildings, plants, and people's clothing were too intense for him to stare at for too long. It was an over-saturation that made his eyes strain with unbearable blindness. His gut felt queasy as if he had eaten too much butter and sugar. As he looked around at the buildings of the past, all haphazardly cobbled together, he couldn't help but feel that this was an arrogant act that defied verboten rules of physics and sensible morality. It was tantamount to a teenage trip to the Gas N' Go, in which Josh would audaciously fill his cup with every soda, mixing them all together into one unholy abomination of sugar and sludge. "Suicide" it was called. And it never tasted good. Or, like when he'd color in his coloring books as a child, mixing all of his favorite crayons together, and while he had hoped they would whorl together to give birth to some extraordinary, undiscovered, new color, perhaps the color to beat all colors, instead the opposite was true: he would be disappointed to find that all it made was a shit brown.

Also, the familiarity of every person and place was profoundly exhausting. At every turn, there was something or someone to remember. Josh was forced to exercise every brain muscle to recognize even the most meaningless face or building structure. Every detail of the city had meaning and purpose. For example, the trees that lined the street were a photocopied version of the single plum tree that sat outside of his grandmother's house. The mailboxes that rested on each corner were made up of the very same mailbox that sat outside of his townhouse in Chicago; he could tell because they had graffiti of cartoon characters that Josh always felt were very funny and creative, engaging in a lewd, sexual act. Even the trash cans, not that there was any trash to be found in this city, but they were the very same trash cans that his family had in their Evanston home, resting underneath the sink.

Then there were the countless people on the street. Every passing stranger was not a stranger at all. He recognized everyone. But similar to the anxiety-inducing environment of a class reunion, Josh had difficulty placing them at first. He'd finally recognize the face, then try to remember the name, then struggle to identify where they sat on the timeline of his life, but before he could connect with them, they'd be gone and replaced with another acquaintance. An old teacher would pass. Then a friend from camp. Then a friend's big brother. Then an elderly neighbor. All from different cities and years and moments of his life.

What's more, they would approach him with exultant familiarity, thus depriving Josh of the standard, comforting buffer of dual parties allowing one another the allotted, social nicety of having the time to reach the same conclusion of who they were and where they knew each other from. This constant bombardment of forced remembrance and organization was mentally taxing. It was a swirling melange of mayhem with incredible detail that had planted seeds of consternation that were beginning to spore within his gut. The specificity of every aspect was cutting into his skull, his head feeling like a blender filled with stained glass, churning and masticating the jagged colors into a liquified slush, swirling them together into an unidentifiable, yet colorful, migraine.

But he was stopped cold when a face appeared that he didn't recognize.

She stood across the street, and she stared back at him. The crowds of buzzing sidewalk patrons rushed by the woman, swerving around her still frame like fish around jutting coral. Her face was pale and bland, no features that stuck out or would be classified as recognizable. She wore a long, black coat and had short, dark hair, which stood out like a stain amongst this world of abrasive color. She was very forgettable, which made her impossible for Josh to place.

She didn't fit anywhere. Not in San Diego, not in Oregon, not in Evanston, not in Chicago. She belonged to nothing. Josh felt immediately relaxed by a face that demanded nothing from him. A welcomed respite, he flashed a smile and waved. She returned the wave, but she did not smile. Josh could not tell whether this woman was foreboding or welcoming, but regardless, she was enthralling.

"Hey, fart face," said Andy. "Why'd you stop moving? Let's go."

"Who is that?"

"Who is who?"

"Her. She," said Josh, pointing. "Who is she?"

Andy stared with Josh at the woman in black, who gazed back at them with phlegmatic coldness. Andy's face turned sour as if sniffing the fetid stench of rotten food. His scowl wore a hint of minatory wariness.

"Oh, forget her, dude," said Andy. "She's weird. I'd stay away."

The crowd around the woman began to bump her. They were hurried citizens on a busy New York street, jostling a stationary tourist. The crowd intensified, pin-balling the woman back and forth until the sea of people had grown into a hulking mass that swallowed her whole. Josh strained to find her, hoping to see her face one last time. But as the crowd cleared, there was no trace of her to be found.

"Holy shit, check out that kick ass car, dude," said Andy, pointing to a muscle car that had just pulled up to the sidewalk.

It was a black Grand Torino with a red racing stripe. It rumbled, guttling gasoline with voracity as it spat clouds of midnight exhaust. It was polished and waxed, glistening on the outside, but it was an absolute beater on the inside. The engine shook underneath the hood like a gremlin trapped inside of a shoebox, fighting the duct-taped lid to break free. Through the windshield, a young woman sat behind the wheel, gently applying dark, purple lipstick in the rearview mirror. Josh immediately recognized the car and its owner from the far reaches of his mind.

"Keira?" he asked no one in particular.

"Who's Keira?" Andy asked.

"Keira Molworsky, the coolest girl ever, man. I can't fucking believe it... I used to have the biggest crush on her all throughout high school. I was obsessed with her, knew everything about her. She smoked Kools, chewed Big Red bubble gum, and wore the same jean jacket every day, even in the summer. That car was a gift from her dad on her sixteenth birthday. She was the first one at school who could drive. That car matched her personality perfectly."

"Did you guys ever date?"

"Yeah, finally. We went on our first date in the fall of senior year. To this day it's the greatest date I've ever been on. I remember it so well, just because it was an amalgamation of everything I was building towards, romantically. I finally got my shot with her."

"You guys fucked?"

"Jesus, Andy," Josh laughed, shrugging off his brackish

comment. "No, nothing physical really happened. I mean, well, I touched her boob."

"Nice!" Andy offered a hand for a low-five, which Josh returned with perfunctory enthusiasm, his ferrous gaze still fixed on the car and the young woman inside.

"Then what happened?"

"We dated. Just until the end of the following summer. She went away to Boston for college, and we fell out of contact. But it was an amazing summer, man. But that date was, and I use this term sincerely, magical, dude."

Josh's smile faded as the flood of memories came rushing back. His visage turned lugubrious as the opaque fog cleared, allowing the grim reality to unfold.

"Something happened to her."

"What happened?"

"She was always edgy, which is what I liked about her. Always pushed things too far, though. But really, she was deeply insecure; we all were at that age, but especially her. Her home life wasn't very good. Her mom was a drunk, and she liked to drink too. We actually used her fake ID to get booze that summer, but it was innocent then. When she went away to Boston, she would call me occasionally, but only when it was really late, and she was fucked up. Then, her voice started to change. I knew how she sounded when she was drunk, she would always slur her words really bad. But it started sounding really loopy, silly, weird. That's when I heard she got into pills. Later, I'm talkin' years later, I heard she kept going and got into heavier stuff. Needles. Someone said they saw her in New York, hanging out with some weird artists, whacked out of her mind, her arms covered in marks. That was the last I heard."

The memory of how things had panned out was so dour, and yet there was the car. A fresh coat of paint and wax, humming and churning as if shocked back to life. The door opened and out she popped. Her hair was pulled back with the exception of one long strand dangling in her face, just how she used to wear it. She wore an acid-wash jean jacket, a choker around her neck, with her nails painted black. She was newly eighteen and was oozing the angst of a kid who couldn't wait to get the fuck out of town. She lit a cigarette, a Kool of course, and Josh watched, amazed, remembering the specific way in which she used to smoke, holding the cigarette as if it were a joint.

"Never too late to go on that date, pal," said Andy, nudging him in the ribs with his elbow.

A drop of rain hit Josh's forehead. Then another. And another. He looked towards the sky and saw a single, portentous rain cloud hovering above him. It was a striking image as it seemed to have formed in an otherwise unblemished sky. It was inky and full, spitting drops down upon him. Josh looked around and found that no one, not even Andy was being rained down upon. He looked up again. Another. And another. And another.

CHAPTER SIX

SALTY TEARS DRIPPED ONTO JOSH'S FACE. THEY splashed onto his cheekbone, clinging to his skin momentarily, pooling until reaching overflow, and snaking down his bruised face in rivulets of tears, down onto his pillow. Steph sedulously dabbed them away with bedside tissue paper, but it was impossible to keep up with the steady, salty rainfall. But these tears did not belong to her.

Raina Worrick, Josh's girlfriend, leaned over him, dramatically sobbing. She stroked his face with the boorish palming of a recent widow, her spasmed breathing and sniffling scoring the movie she believed she was starring in. Her maudlin facial performance was Oscar-worthy as it contorted like the eponymous masks of the theater.

She yammered routine comforts, "I'm here now, baby," and "It's okay, it's going to be alright," and the one that made Steph cringe the most, the obligatory, "Mama's here, now. Mama's got you."

"Was that a nickname you agreed upon?" asked Steph through gritted teeth.

"My poor baby," said Raina, continuing without hearing her. "My poor, poor Joshua."

Josh-ua? Steph's massive eye roll upon hearing her brother's full name nearly sent her tumbling backward. Raina had revealed herself to be a fraud at that very moment. No one called him Joshua. Only Grammy Jan called him Joshua, and he would always blush and cringe when she said it. He was a Josh, through and through.

"I always told him to wear a helmet," she cried. "I always told him..."

"Mhm. How long have you guys been dating?" Steph asked, pointedly, sounding like her mother.

"Five months. But it feels like it could be five years."

Raina was short and blonde, though Steph could tell by her exposed roots that this was not her natural hair color. She was from Hinsdale, a wealthy Chicago suburb. Her skin was soaked in tanning spray, her lips caked with a pink gloss, she wore yoga pants and the sweatshirt of her college alma mater. She looked like a rejected Barbie doll: Illinois Suburbs Barbie. Steph never got along with these girls, and she failed to see what Josh saw in Raina. They had gone out for drinks after work one night when the two had first started dating. Raina was constantly on her phone, chronicling the evening on Instagram and texting one of her friends who apparently was "going through a really hard time right now." When Raina left to take a call from her friend to "talk her off a ledge," Steph asked what Josh saw in her.

"I've never dated a stereotypical 'hot girl' before," he replied. "And this is my opportunity."

Steph felt rare repulsion, one of the only times she had ever felt that way towards her brother.

"How could you be so shallow?" she asked, again sounding like her mother.

"It's only temporary, Sis," he said, assuring her. "I know, trust me, I see it too."

Steph smiled as Raina returned to the table. "Oh my god, my friend is a total wreck," said Raina, taking her seat and unconvincingly suppressing her tears. There was an awkward silence as she waited for someone to ask her what was going on.

"What's going on?" asked Steph, now hoping to provoke the reaction she was expecting, a pedantic regaling of a meaningless and bland breakup. Steph thought she caught the beginning of a smirk in the corner of Raina's mouth as if she were thankful for the opportunity to perform.

"It's the one-year anniversary of her boyfriend of two years breaking up with her," said Raina, overcome with maudlin emotion. "Now, he just posted a picture with another girl, and she looks exactly like her. So she's totally freaking out. And then, she saw on his Instagram story that he went to a..."

Steph could feel her focus fading as she slowly tuned Raina out and looked to Josh, who was doing the same. They smiled at one another, that same smile they shared in the back seat of their parent's Volvo station wagon in the midst of a long road trip when Mom or Dad would say something stupid about a modern song that came on the radio, a hatred for a current fashion trend, or genuine befuddlement concerning reality television. They'd share this very same wry smile; the invisible, taut line of sarcastic sibling connection.

Here Raina was, putting on a show for no one. Her mascara ran like her eyes were melting, decorative candles; black wax trickling down her face. Steph cringed as every maudlin tear fell onto Josh's cheek. She felt as if they were drops of poison, inimical to his health. She diligently dabbed them away.

"Maybe you should sit down, Raina," said Steph. "Like, away from Josh for a minute. Give him some air."

"Right, right," she said, baffled and overwhelmed. She crossed to the chairs against the wall, slumping into one and dropping her head into her hands. "What are the doctors saying?" she asked. "Did they do a head scan?"

"A CAT Scan? Yes."

"Well, what did it say? Is he brain dead?!"

"No, no. It came back negative for blocked arteries, and they've seen little to no swelling. His Glasgow Ranking is a seven, which is a fairly deep coma. It ranges from three to fifteen, three being deep, fifteen being wakeable. So they're putting him on nutrients-"

"Oh my god, he's being fed through a tube?"

"No. IV nutrients for the next couple weeks while they monitor his brain functionality. They've tested various stimuli, but haven't seen any results. They've managed to determine that he's about nine percent conscious, so they're trying different things to pull him further out. The good news is, they see robust brain activity. So, that's very good."

Raina was immediately overwhelmed by the debriefing, which is what Steph wanted. She popped up, pacing, rubbing her face with her hands. She was living in a nebulous nightmare that she couldn't shake her way out of. Steph could see her going through the math in her head, miscalculating everything. Finally, she stopped. Her knees buckled as she fell to the floor. She knelt, tackled by grief, looking towards the sky, which was the ceiling.

"Why? Why Lord? Why him?" she asked, whispering in desperate supplication.

Who was this performance for? Steph thought. Surely

not Josh. Was it for her? Maybe it was for the passing nurses? Was it for an imaginary audience? No matter who it was for, one thing became excruciatingly clear: Raina lacked self-awareness to the point of being oblivious to the fact that her one-act play was not being well received by any audience, real or imaginary. Steph felt the bubble of simmering rage in her stomach as she watched Raina's performance crescendo.

"He was so young! We had so many plans," she cried.

"What took you so long to get here?" asked Steph with piercing asperity.

"Excuse me?" Raina asked, snapping to, her Shakespearean character evaporating before her eyes.

"I called you two days ago. I left a couple of messages. What took you so long to get here?" Steph stared at her with bare coldness, hoping to make the air as frigid as possible. It worked as Raina rose to her feet, squirming like a nightcrawler on a hook.

"I... I couldn't bring myself to look at him. The thought... of him lying here in this bed by himself..."

"He wasn't by himself. We were all here."

"I know, I know. I'm just not... I'm not as strong as you guys. You have to understand."

"Oh, I understand. Believe me, I understand."

"It's just that," said Raina, scrambling and stopping short. Steph enjoyed watching the rat fumble its way through the maze, aimlessly wandering in a starved panic, hoping that the next turn would reveal an exit. "Joshua and I, ya know, we had a very special connection."

"You mean 'have,' right? You 'have' a very special connection."

"Right! Have. We have..."

"After five months."

Raina returned Steph's glowering now, deciding to

square off with her. Steph did everything she could not to blink, even though one eye felt severely dry. She finally succumbed, but only slightly, bringing one eyelid down to refresh it. But this caused her confrontational stare to morph into a slow half-wink, which had a more significant impact that could have ever been assumed. It came off as a rude gesture of aggressive panache. Raina folded, averting her gaze, and moving to Josh's side again.

"It's okay, Joshua. I'm here, baby," she said, stroking his hair. She went to fluff his pillow but stopped as she inspected it. "These are much too hard for him, Stephanie. He has a head injury, after all."

Raina yanked the pillow from underneath Josh and ran into the hallway, flagging down a nurse. "Excuse me! My boyfriend needs another pillow! Something softer, this one is much too hard."

The nurse looked confused. "I'm sorry, miss, we only have one kind of-"

"Just get him a different one! I can't deal with the thought of him being uncomfortable. He needs to feel... he needs to be..." Her chest started to spasm again as her breathing became rapid and tight, betokening a crying fit. Tears finally came, pouring from the corners of her eyes, and the nurse quickly nodded and ran off to retrieve a different pillow to appease her.

Steph had tolerated this ridiculous show for long enough, and she had only done so because it was cloistered away, confined to this room where it couldn't hurt anyone. But now, Raina's voracious need for attention was spilling out into the world. Steph seethed, forming the sentences of reproach that would start with, "Why don't you go fuck yourself?"

As if on cue, Lisa and Rich shuffled into the room.

"Raina," said Rich with a warm smile. "You made it."

Raina rushed into his arms, relieved to see him as if Rich had just returned from war. He enveloped her in a warm hug, gently patting her back as she sobbed into his chest. Steph was confused and enraged.

"You guys have met?"

"Of course," said Lisa. "Josh brought her over for Sunday dinner a few months ago."

"A few months ago?" asked Steph. "They had been dating for a couple months, and Josh thought that was long enough to bring her to Sunday dinner?"

"Well, you would have known that if Sunday dinner remained a priority," said Lisa.

Steph fumed as she thought back on Josh's promise of Raina and his relationship being "only temporary." You don't invite a temporary partner to meet Lisa Husk. She felt the sting of betrayal from her sibling beyond his unconsciousness.

"How are you holding up, dear?" Lisa asked Raina.

"Not well, Mrs. Husk. Not well at all. I just can't bear to see him like this."

"I know. It's terrible."

"I'm sorry I didn't come sooner. I just couldn't bear it."

"We're all on our own timeline, dear. I understand."

Who was this example of empathy and altruism who had materialized before her, Steph thought. Where was her caustic, biting mother?

"He's just so full of life, you know?" said Raina. "He always has something funny to say, or he's running all over the place, always heading somewhere. And to see him lying in this bed like this..."

Lisa sniffled, letting out a small whimper, which brought the room to a standstill. The air was vacuumed from the space as all eyes fell on the traditionally stoic matriarch as she began to crumble. It was like watching the cracking and crumbling of an impregnable fortress, having finally succumbed to an enemy onslaught.

Rich became alarmed by his wife's weakened state. At first, he didn't know whether or not it was real. He couldn't remember the last time he saw her cry. He strained to remember. She didn't cry when her mother died; or when either child was born. She most certainly didn't cry on their wedding day. It finally came to him. It had been somewhere around twenty years ago. She had been working on the house all day, gardening in the morning and cleaning the kitchen in the afternoon. It was summer, she was exhausted and hot, and she stubbed her toe on the coffee table. This was also the last time he heard her swear.

"Shit!" she screamed.

"Are you okay?" he had asked.

She didn't answer. She bit her lip as tears rolled down her face. Rich was shocked.

"Lisa. Dear, are you crying? What's the matter?"

She grabbed her car keys and left the house. He heard the Volvo start and pull out of the driveway. She returned three hours later, after dinner, and refused to speak of it.

Steph fumed as she watched Raina's bullshit corrode her mother's composure. It was a dam Lisa had spent decades erecting, only to succumb to an act of emotional terrorism. Steph had no clue what to do, no idea how to help. She had never seen her like this. Lisa squeaked like a whimpering church mouse, doing her best to hide her face. Steph inched closer, resting her hand on her shoulder, which Lisa quickly shrugged off.

Steph felt ostracized as she watched Rich hold Raina and Lisa, both crying in his arms. She couldn't help but take in the image of them as if they were a separate, familial unit, posing for a portrait that Steph was taking. What fomented her apoplexy further was that the image seemed to work. They made a convincing family.

"I'll never forget our first date," said Raina, unprompted as she wafted to Josh's bedside, making a meal of her movement, sponging up the room's bleak scenery. She stared intensely into Josh's vacant expression.

"He took me to Navy Pier. We walked along the water, holding hands. He was so polite, so sweet. I had never been with someone so kind. We played a few carnival games. He won me a small bear from the ring toss. I still have it, somewhere. Finally, we rode the Ferris Wheel. I guess he had told the ride operator to stop it at the top, which was where he asked if he could kiss me. It was so romantic. Then, he took me to dinner at his favorite Italian restaurant: Buca di Beppo."

Steph snorted, laughter bubbling out of her. As the alternate family stared at her, she quickly quashed her chortling.

"I'm sorry. That sounds really sweet."

She laughed again, unable to bury it.

"A tourist trap and a national restaurant chain," she muttered. "Nice going, Josh."

Raina threw a virulent stare.

"Sorry, Raina," said Steph. "Continue. I'm eager to hear the rest."

"As I was saying, he was such a gentleman. A very special guy. I saw a real future for us. Marriage, a house, children, all of it. It pains me to think that it all may be lost now."

"You guys met on a dating app, right?" asked Steph, her temerity slicing through Raina's performance.

Lisa gave Steph a minatory stare, but it softened quickly. Her icy blue eyes had melted to a weak twinkle. Steph was surprised and disappointed. As if she were suddenly aware of her exhaustion, Lisa slumped into a nearby chair and heaved a sigh of resignation. Steph could see her reeling; all of the grim possibilities running through her head. This only stoked her flames of hatred towards Raina.

"My poor Joshua," said Raina, caressing his head.

"My mother called him by his full name," said Lisa.

"Mom?" asked Steph, gently. There was no reply.

"Lisa," Rich firmly offered up, hoping to prod her out of her trance.

Lisa gently looked up to no one in particular, her jaw hanging open. She looked dumbfounded by the chaos, her eyes were glassy and empty. Finally, she sought Rich for help, a fighter hoping for their corner to throw in the towel.

"How about we go home and have some lunch?" Rich asked. "What do you say, Lees?"

She slowly nodded, zombified. Rich helped her to her feet, he clutching to her and she to him. As they drifted towards the door, Lisa jolted to life.

"Stephanie. If you hear of any updates, please-"

"I'll call you, Mom."

Lisa nodded and looked to Josh, taking in his frangible state one last time before Rich delicately ushered her out of the room. Steph's eyes remained on the doorway even after they had gone. She barely noticed that Raina had begun to pace the room again.

"Oh my god, that was so sad," said Raina. "Your poor mother is an absolute wreck."

"Mhm," mumbled Steph, reticent and heavy.

Gone was Raina's widowed character, replaced now by toilsome anxiety, her skin feeling irritated by her bleak surroundings.

"God, I hate hospitals," said Raina as she itched. "There's so much bad shit that happens here, and it's all happening at once. It's so freaky, man."

The concept of mortality was winding her up, as if a tornado of transient awareness had enveloped her, spinning her around on the waxy, linoleum floor. Her head was twirling as her eyes darted around the room, suddenly conscious of her confining space.

"Last year, I almost died," she said. "I was driving on the highway, and I was going to change lanes and this guy two lanes over, he decides to change lanes at the exact same time. And I just didn't see him. We came within inches of one another. Like, really, inches. It was so scary. And he was in a big SUV, and I was in my little Fiat. He would have just torn right through me. I avoided the highway for like, a month after that."

Steph watched her now. For the first time, this was not a performance. Raina's spinning-out felt unfeigned. Steph's hatred for her had ceased. She was overcome with pity for poor Raina. She watched as Raina hurriedly paced, back and forth, back and forth. Finally, she stopped, an idea coming to her.

"Maybe I should grab everyone something to eat," offered Raina.

"Sure," said Steph.

"Or, maybe not food, but like, magazines or something."

"Sounds great," said Steph, nodding with understanding.

"If I left, would you be cool by yourself? It's just, now that I'm thinking about it, I have a few errands I need to run. But I can try to grab some dinner and come back. Magazines, too. What kind do you like? Is that okay? Steph? Can I go? Does that work?"

"You can go, Raina."

Raina sighed with relief, then was hit with a burst of optimism. "I'll be back in a little while. You want pizza? Or a burger, maybe? Is *People Magazine* okay?"

"Sure."

"Great. I'll totally be right back. Well, I kinda have to... I have to drive... I'm going to head to my sisters," she said, garrulous and erratic. "I have to stop by there. And then... I have some other things. Some laundry. But I'll grab some pizza. I'll let you low if I'm running late. Or if I can't make it back."

"Sure, that sounds great."

Raina rushed to her purse, collecting her things quickly. She did a quick inspection, frazzled, but making sure she had everything. She darted for the door but stopped.

"I'll be right back."

"Go ahead. It's okay."

"Probably two hours. Maybe three."

"Okay. Go ahead."

She started to leave but stopped again.

"I'll text you if I can't make it back for some reason."

"Okay. Thank you, Raina."

They shared a smile and Raina slipped out the door, not even giving Josh a final glimpse. After a moment of silence, the door opened again. Steph was startled at first, thinking she had said goodbye to someone she would never see again. She was proven to be correct as the person who entered the room was the nurse that Raina had demanded bring Josh a new pillow.

"Someone asked for this," the nurse said, awkwardly.

"Oh, yes. We did."

The nurse moved to the bed to change Josh's pillow, but Steph stopped her.

"No, that's okay. He's fine. Just leave that here with me."

The nurse, confused for a moment, finally shrugged and handed it over and left. Steph inspected the pillow and rolled her eyes. She threw it aside. But as she did, she was hit with a moment of curiosity. She examined Josh's pillow, which felt like any standard pillow. Then she felt the one the nurse had brought. There was no difference. Or, maybe there was. She felt the pillow lying under his head again. This time she felt more feathers. It was somewhat prickly, spiny. This was in contrast to the pillow that the nurse had brought, which was a little smoother and seemed to have no feathers at all.

She switched the pillows out. She lifted his head with tender care, removing the, perhaps, overly-feathered pillow, and replacing it with the maybe softer, more cushioned pillow. Or, at least she thought so. Who's to say for sure.

While she debated the difference between the pillows, she carefully caressed his head, running her fingers through his hair.

CHAPTER SEVEN

You GENTLY MOVE YOUR HAND THROUGH YOUR HAIR, staring into the mirror with conviction. Today is the beginning of the life you've been building towards. Your adult life begins now. It's Sunday, a renowned holy day, and although you don't believe in that malarkey, it still feels sacred. As if created and shaped by the divine, this has the makings of the perfect day. The best, and first, day of your life.

You've taken every precaution in your preparation. You bought and used a new body wash, which you chose with careful consideration. You had sifted through the soaps, sniffing and evaluating their masculine scents as if you were wine tasting in Burgundy, finally arriving at one which gave off a proper concoction of the robust scents of testosterone and elegance. Having lathered up and caked your skin with it, it has fermented with your budding pheromones to produce a scented aura that makes you feel as if you were a well-read lumberjack. It gives you the confidence to bullfight. If you were in Spain, having just soaked yourself in this particular body wash, you feel as though you would descend the steps of a coliseum, leaping into the arena, and shoving the bedizened, denizen fighter out of your way. The bull, now your adversary, would be distracted by your cavalier confidence. It would suffer a severe lack of confidence and buckle, slinking away in cowardice. The crowd would roar. Your muscles would flex in triumph.

You are mighty.

But you have to be sure. This is the date you've been waiting for, after all. You can't risk going with only one scent. That's why you've stolen your father's aftershave. You actually did manage to shave, getting rid of that detestable peach fuzz that your mother always hated and made comments about.

"It makes you look dirty. You have such a pretty face, why don't you let people see it?!"

You splash the aftershave onto your palms and rub it onto your lithesome cheeks. "Yowza!" you say, just like Dad. It doesn't burn, but you know it should. Maybe it does. Perhaps you can feel it a little bit. You can. Definitely. You're a man.

You've also managed to sneak his cologne. It's a small bottle that he only uses for special occasions; holiday parties, super bowl gatherings, dinners with Mom's family. You spray two squirts onto each wrist and rub them into your jaw. But again, it doesn't feel like enough.

Cursed be the creator who made it impossible to sniff thine own self!

You take the extra precaution and spray the scent onto your shirt, six squirts. Now you can successfully smell the melange of pungent masculinity that you've concocted. This is a brawny aura that could make Paul Bunyon weep, and Rocky Balboa take a dive.

As you put on your sneakers, you feel as though you've done all that you can do. You've gone that extra mile. Your sneakers are an iridescent white after vigorously scrubbing them with the white sneaker cleaner that you bought at the shoe outlet. They sparkle and shine like pearly whale's teeth. You put on your watch. You want the world at large to know that you're a man who needs to adhere to time. You're a man with a schedule and demands. You're a man who has places to be and problems to solve. It was the watch Grammy Jan got you for Christmas last year, and she totally fucking nailed it. It's far too big for your tiny wrist, but you are convinced that this is stylish - it's what so many of the rappers in music videos wear; a man bracelet that will convince her you are wealthy, or well on your way. This is bound to impress.

Every box being checked in your auspicious preparation, you climb into your old pickup truck. It's a massive, brown, extended cab with four-wheel drive. It's fifteen-years-old with a hundred and fifty miles on it. It slurps up fossil fuels as if it had a twisty straw stabbed into the earth's crust. It's not the most glamorous chariot, but it's certainly passable considering your age. It was a gift from your grandparents, half-burden/half-reward for making the honor roll throughout middle school and the amount of high school you've currently experienced. In preparation for the date of a lifetime, you had your crack windshield replaced and freon added to the air conditioning so you and Keira wouldn't sweat through your clothes, as you were sure to perspire today.

You drive, your gut stewing with unwieldy anxiety. After years of planning, it was all coming to fruition. It began with jokes two years ago in Biology. You were new to town, having moved from Oregon. Evanston, Illinois was bigger than the town you had just come from. It felt like a city! What's-more, it was outside of one of the biggest cities in the United States: Chicago, baby. And Evanston itself had a different vibe. The kids had more money. There were fast food restaurants here. The high school was three-times the size of your puny Oregon school. You knew you had to make your mark somehow, so you used humor. You quickly garnered a reputation as a precocious wisecracker. Not a class clown by any means, but a nettlesome classroom disturbance who offered mordant asides to his classmates at the expense of the syllabus.

As your reputation and confidence grew, you began to focus your targeting. What began as a wide net of classroom commentary began to focus and become play-by-play asides to a section of the room, more specifically where Keira Molworsky sat. As the year went on, your jokes were sequestered to the lab table that you shared with Keira and four others. Soon, by year's end, there were whispered wisecracks to Keira alone. The following years, a spirited friendship had blossomed. What classes you managed to have with her, you made sure you sat as close as possible. The flirting was usually subtle, always disguised as caustic comments, but underneath burned an intense love for this girl.

Finally, senior year came, and you both had leadership together. Thank your mother's Lord Almighty for leadership, the poor man's free period. You and Keira were often paired together to work on projects and fundraisers. You were tasked with helping run a campaign to increase recycling efficiency at the school, which to you felt tantamount to the team building experience of a husband and wife renovating a house. And it was here that you got the one-on-one time that you yearned for so desperately. Intimate conversations were had. She told you everything: her mom drinks too much, she always wanted to go to Italy, her older sister moved to Austin, Texas, and she visited there a couple times, and it's the coolest city in the world. You debated movies, music, and the purpose of homework. And on top of it all, you made an excellent team, seemingly conquering every task with ease. You managed to raise three-hundred and forty-two dollars for homecoming from recycled materials from the lunch room. You were heroes.

As a result of your efficiency, Mrs. Lund always paired you two up on every task. Finally, when you mustered the courage to ask her to hang out over the weekend, it felt like all but a guarantee. You'd betray the demands of nature if you denied your passion for one another. You were working on a banner for the Pep Rally, Keira doing the handwriting because yours was atrocious. And you just asked her. Point blank. It came fumbling out of your mouth. And you paused, terrified. What if you were wrong? What if she hated you all along and was just being nice to you? What if this was some ruse? She was just nice to you out of pity, you fool! But it was too late, you had already asked her. You watched her stop her marker midway through scrawling. She lifted her beautiful face, her cheeks turning pink as she flashed you a smile. It was the smile you always worked so hard to achieve. The trophy for every dumb joke. And boy did you melt. You were a puddle on that floor, man.

"Yeah. Sure," she said.

Holy shit. Now you were both grinning like idiots as you returned to your work, blithely ignoring the apparent epochal shift; acting as if the atmosphere around you hadn't changed. As if everything weren't going to be different from now on. And just like that, the date of your dreams had a green light.

You're too eager. You're on track to be forty-five minutes early. You adapt. You slow down to a crawl of twenty-five miles per hour. Good move. You want to savor "the moment before." You drive through the neighborhood streets, observing the houses you've never taken the time to appreciate. They were beautiful cookie-cutter homes with people going about their day like this was any other normal Sunday.

You're burning too much gas. You don't want to have to stop to fill-up during your date, you'll look like an ill-prepared stooge. You have to park. So you do, down the block from her house. You do your best to kill a half hour, fiddling with the radio, staring at the clock. You flip over to AM and listen to sports radio. You stare into the distance as the AM fuzz engulfs you in static. A fog of purgatory. Three o'clock is on its way. It's coming. It's inevitable. If only you could will it. You should have made it for two o'clock! You'd already be on your date! You make a decision: fuck it. You're going to be fifteen minutes early. Who gives a shit? So you'll come off too eager, who cares? You care, but you tell yourself you don't.

As you coast up to her parent's gorgeous two-story house, a house so perfect it is emulous of the girl you are hopelessly in love with, she comes floating out the front door. It really is a perfect house, one that you hope to see the inside of some-day. You imagine the staircase to be rich mahogany. It looks particularly festive during the holidays, festooned with garlands and white lights (a tasteful selection compared to the multicolored strands, of course). The stairs lead to her bedroom, which is filled with posters of the bands you both love but also embarrassing remnants of her past.

You'll ask questions about them, "Is that a Cabbage Patch Kid?!" And she'll defend herself by saying she couldn't bear to part with it. You'll meet her parents. "Hello, I'm Josh. I'm the man who will father your grandchildren. Can I use your bathroom?" Mr. Molworsky will shake your hand and say, "I admire the confidence, young man. You remind me of myself. The bathroom is behind the stairs to the right. Take your time."

If everything goes well today, this dream will become a reality.

As she bounds off the porch, she hovers above the ground as she drifts towards your truck like a lovely apparition. You open the door for her like a true gentleman. She hoists herself into the passenger seat with ease and grace. She's wearing a sundress, black boots, and her jean jacket. She's ready for everything.

"You look great," you say, your voice quavering. Your throat feels like it's closing up, reacting as if you have a terrible shellfish allergy.

"You too. I love your cologne," she says, smiling. A moment of silence between you as you sit in the truck. Holy fuck, are you guys going to kiss now? Already?? No. Instead, she gives you a swift punch in the arm. She laughs and winks. Amazing.

As you drive, she fiddles with the radio, making herself comfortable. She puts her boots up on the dash. Immediately, she has made this truck her own, and you love it.

"So, what do you wanna do?" she asks.

You were expecting this. You have a plan. You reach under the seat and pull out a small liquor bottle, a bottle of rum; 151, to be exact. The heavy, serious stuff. You hate your part-time job, working at a small grocery store, but it has its occasional perks. Pete, the weird/old checker, was one of them. You asked him to buy the liquor for you. He agreed with an eery smile as if you had just sold him your soul. One of the subjects you bonded over with Keira was drinking. Not that you did any, but she made it sound as if she did, so you mirrored her experiences with tall-tales of your own. She said she used to steal gin from her mother's liquor cabinet and replace it with water. She'd sneak into the garage and raid her father's beer fridge and take them over to her friend's houses.

When she'd ask you about drinking you'd lie, filling your weekends with fantastic fables of alcohol-induced debauchery.

"Why didn't I see you at so-and-so's party?" she'd ask.

The reason was obvious: you were either not invited or didn't have the balls to defy your parents and sneak out. Instead, you'd fastidiously parry with a badass excuse.

"I don't like parties. They make me too anxious. I'd rather just drink by myself," you'd say. What a load of crap, but she seemed to buy it. You came across as troubled, messed up, deep.

"Cool," she'd say. "I get it."

But the portrait you had painted her, that of a fledged drinker with the sangfroid of a kid from the wrong side of the tracks, had given yourself unrealistic expectations of alcohol tolerance. What did this imaginary, troubled young man drink? You had no fucking clue. So you decided to go with the hardest stuff imaginable: 151, the stuff that could pull paint off of a warplane. You based this off of stories Pete told you on his breaks. They always involved him "blacking out" and causing a scene at his ex-girlfriend's house. Pete was super weird. This was sure to work.

But when you offered her the bottle, she gave you a polite, surprising rebuke.

"Nah, I have homework. If it was Saturday, then for sure."

Well, now you're totally fucked. So much for the perfect date! You're such an idiot. Why didn't you think of that?! Of course, she has homework! So do you! The date is a disaster. You'll never see the inside of her house. Her parents would hate you anyway. Keira needs a man full of ideas, and you're such an empty-headed fuck they won't even let you come inside, let alone see the girl's room! "Get the fuck out of my house, young man," Mr. Molworsky would probably say. This seals it: you're going to die alone.

You calm yourself down. She hasn't opened the door and decided to tuck-and-roll. She seems to be willing to play it by ear. You wrack your brain, searching for an idea. The movies! This was also a frequent topic of conversation between you two. And the movie theater is dark, which could lead to making out, at the very least holding hands. Yes, this could work.

"We could do a movie," you offer up.

"Sure," she says, nonchalant.

She is either completely over this date, or doesn't care what you do because she's just happy to be on this date. Dear god are you hoping it's the latter.

But trouble strikes again as you get to the movie theater and you can't decide on a movie. There's the comedy with that big comedian from SNL. He always does those weird, broad characters. This might be his most over-the-top yet: he gets mistaken for an astronaut and sent to space. One of the previews had a bit where he farts in the cockpit, and no one can escape it. You happen to like his movies, but they're notoriously panned as low-brow. You'll see it later, but that's out for now. Then there's the action movie with the buff, bald dude. A plane, that is also flying city, gets hijacked by terrorists. He just retired, but he's the only man who can land the flying metropolis. This one promises to be excellent, but you're scared that you'll look like a cliche guy if you choose that movie.

"I'd rather not do that one," you say. "There's not enough strong, female characters."

She throws you a surprised expression, skeptical, but finally nods in agreement. Then there's the romantic drama with that guy who parts his hair in the middle and lets strands of it dangle in his face. He's a soldier in World War II and is injured in battle, but saved by a French widow. She nurses him back to health, but trouble arises when she learns that he has a wife back home. Will he stay? Which love will he choose? She says that she could see that one, but you're intimidated. What if she falls in love with this guy and decides that you don't add up? This is supposed to be the best day of your life, not his. Back off, silver-screen lothario!

As you debate movie choices, you can feel the date slipping through your fingers. You panic.

"How about we just go get some coffee?" she suggests.

Brilliant. Coffee.

"Yes!" you say too loudly. "I love coffee!"

You've never had coffee. You don't know what the fuck you're talking about. I mean, you've had a sip from your dad's mug, but you were like, nine or something. And you despised it. It was bitter and gross, tasting like sour soil water. Disgusting. What if you ordered a coffee and upon sipping it, you spit it out? She'd know that you were a fraud. A lier! She'd connect the dots, realizing that you've been lying about everything you told her. You were nothing more than a sham.

She held your hand.

Gasp! Just like that. It catches you off guard. Weren't you supposed to do that? This doesn't make any sense, but it doesn't matter because it is happening and it is glorious. Her skin! Her hand is soft and smooth. Warm and small, delicate. The muscles of her hands are made of marshmallows or the foam of those mattresses that mold to your frame. Of course, she has perfect hands! And she tucks her thumb into your palm, a strange quirk that you instantly fall in love with. Holy hell you can do this forever. You each say nothing as you stroll, taking your time, enjoying the moment. You will drink all of the shitty soil water in the world for this girl.

At the coffee shop, you stand in line, holding hands. You have a tacit agreement not to let go, doing everything you can to remain in contact. If you let go, who knows when you'll get it back? You each order a coffee, hers with extra almond milk. You order yours black because you think it makes you more masculine. You're a man who knows what he wants. A man of simple needs. A straight shooter.

It tastes awful, but not as bad as you expected. You can hang with this.

You and Keira walk along the sidewalk, holding hands. You pass a nearby park and decide to venture in. For once, you're not scrambling in search of a plan. This is perfect in and of itself. It's fall in Illinois. It's an imperturbable paradise of deciduous beauty. The leaves have morphed into a burnt ochre. A slight breeze whips through the trees, creating a gentle susurrus. The air is thin and cold, but the sun is warm. It's a perfect balance of every texture and temperature.

Keira finds a spot on the grass on a slanting hillside. A game of "kick the can" is in progress for a kid's birthday party. You both watch the game in silence, still clasping hands, feeling as if it has aged your relationship into an elderly married couple. Your hands caress each other, dancing. Your hands are totally having sex, you think. She uses her mani-cured nails to gingerly scratch the inside of your forearm, leading into the palm of your hand. It's an affectionate gesture that gives you butterflies in your stomach.

You talk about the future. Graduation. College. After college. Places you'll visit. Who you'll become. What career you'll have. You say that you'll be a video game developer. Maybe you'll be on the forefront of the creation of virtual reality. Regardless, it will be in computers. Something amazing and incredible. You'll make a boatload of money and buy a big house in the northwest. She's never been. You tell her that it's wet, green, and beautiful. You'll buy your dream car, a '57 Coupe Deville. But you'll also have a Honda or something; a vehicle that is energy efficient because, you know, you care about the planet and you also want to stay grounded.

She's going to be a music producer, which makes sense because she knows everything about music. The coolest job for the coolest person. She wants to help bands formulate their sound. She wants to be cutting edge. She wants to help make music that changes the world. She wants to work in New York City, specifically in the Empire State Building. She wants to travel everywhere for her job, meeting all kinds of artists and people. And she'll do it, too. You know she will.

You walk back to your truck, hands delicately wrestling with one another. You've thrown away your coffee, managing to drink a third of it. But now you're jittery as hell, and your breath reeks. Oh god. Your lack of preparation has struck again. Well, if you were expecting a kiss now, you better forget it! You fucking dumb ass! You should have planned for this!

Just then, she whips out a pack of Big Red gum, her signature brand. She unwraps a piece and places it in her mouth. She notices you staring and offers you a piece. What a lifesaver. A kiss is still within the realm of possibility.

As you get into the truck, you make a decision. You ditch the gum. This is happening. As you climb in, you notice that she's done the same. Oh god, is this really happening? Maybe you should drive her back home and do it there. That's when it happens, right? At the end of the date? As you shut the door, you put the keys in the ignition, but something stops you. It's the ideal time.

You go in for the kiss.

Your kissing history has been riddled with failure. Your

first was when you were thirteen. Julie Starsovich. And you were absolutely terrible. It happened under the bleachers during a football game. You didn't know what to do with your tongue, having been instructed by well-regarded Ladies Man and mathematics colleague, Frank "Boner" Bonerro. Boner told you to slide your tongue in and out of the girl's mouth. As a result, you stabbed your tongue into poor Julie's mouth like a predatory eel erupting from a cave in search of reef prey. Just really, really bad.

Your second experience was with Amanda Weest when you were fourteen. This was in the hallway during lunch. She was very brazen, forcefully pressing you into your locker. You had learned from your failure with Julie that you had to be more delicate. Movies had taught you that the tongue needed to roll more, the gratuitous silhouettes in that one 80's fighter pilot movie being a prime example. So you tried this thing where you pressed the tip of your tongue behind your front teeth, then rolled the tongue out with a slow flop. It felt like you were a trained whale that was unfurling its tongue from its mouth, awaiting a fish. Awful, just awful. The third was Michelle Camillo, sophomore year. This was at Gabby Miller's birthday party where you played Seven Minutes in Heaven. You decided to follow Michelle's lead on this one, but it turned out that she was no better a kisser than you. It morphed into strange jawing with tongues touching outside of your mouths. Mostly just a bunch of heavy breathing into each other's faces. You clacked teeth at one point. It was more profoundly confusing than anything.

You were worried that you'd be a disappointment to Keira, but this was not so. She was so supportive. She was on a whole other planet. Her lips delicately pressed into yours like an old-fashioned movie kiss, the ones in black and white where the men wore trench coats and said "sweetheart," and it wasn't douchey. She used almost no tongue, and when she did, it was sparingly deployed and welcomed. It was a soft, gentle kiss. Suddenly, she used her nose, bumping yours ever so slightly, nuzzling like an adorable mammal from the Arctic. Holy hell was she good at this.

You get an idea. You aren't proud of it, but it just pops into your head.

Do you grab her boob?

You weigh your options: this kiss is going so amazingly well, maybe you just enjoy it. But then again, you've dreamed of this. You've always wondered what they felt like. But what if you offend her? What if she pulls away and slaps you?

You venture your hand north but pause. You decide against it, retreating. But as she turns, pulling you closer for a different kissing angle, your hand happens to fall on it. It's there, and it wasn't your call! Purely organic! You give two gentle squeezes. You're in heaven.

Then, you pull your hand away. This isn't all about her boobs, man! Focus.

People walk by the truck, staring into the windshield at your gross display of teenage affection, rolling their eyes. They look either jealous or disgusted. Who knows. Fuck 'em! The fools, they could not possibly fathom the importance of this kiss.

You part, but your faces stay close. You can feel her breath, warm and inviting. Her eyelids are heavy, eyes soft.

"What took you so long?" she asks.

"I don't know," you hear yourself say.

On the drive back to her house, you hold hands in silence. You each wear a guilty grin as if you've managed to pull off some major bank heist. You wish this day would never end, time submitting to your unreasonable desire and allowing you to exist in this moment for eternity.

You pull up to her house, and neither of you can bear to move. Then, deciding to succumb to the inevitability, she opens the door and hops out. She smiles, her visage perfectly framed by her light brown hair. She walks towards her house. You watch her, fondly. But suddenly, she stops halfway. She comes jogging back. Why is she coming back? You look around in the truck, thinking that maybe she's forgotten something. She opens the door, hopping back in, and kissing you once more. Passionately and delicately.

"Just wanted one more," she says.

On the way home, you drive around the block. Your heart races and your adrenaline wreaks havoc on your nervous system. You can't calm down. You're unwilling to pull into your driveway because if you do, then the day will end. The night will come, bringing tomorrow with it, and today will be nothing more than a fond memory. It slips like sand through the creases of your hands. You want to bask in the glow of the moment for as long as you can until it is unquestionably gone.

You finally park, shutting off the truck. You sit, staring out into the street, recounting everything that happened. Beat by beat. You can't forget one modicum of this day. Your heart still races, pounding on the wall of your sternum. You watch as an old couple walks their dog, holding hands like you had just done a few hours ago. You watch as the old couple converse, the old man motioning towards one of the houses they're walking past. He's probably commenting on the shoddy roofing job. Or how unkempt the grass is. Or how the gutters are full of leaves. You think, maybe that will be us one day. Or maybe not. Maybe they have no idea what this feeling is. Does anyone?

CHAPTER EIGHT

"Fuck, I'm sorry I'm late," said Shawn Koehler, rushing into the hospital room. Steph sat in a chair against the wall, head leaned back as if she had been sleeping.

"Late?" asked Steph. "I wasn't expecting you at any specific time."

"I know, but still. I texted you, and I said I'd be here an hour ago, but the fucking line at McDonald's was fucking huge. It was a total shit show."

Shawn stopped, frozen as he took Josh in for the first time. His casual demeanor melted, replaced by shock and terror.

"Jesus..."

He stood, jaw agape as if he'd been stung by a stiff jab. His brow contorted, struggling with what to do with the grim image.

"Yeah. He's actually doing better," said Steph. "Or at least, better than he was."

Shawn tried to hide his uneasiness, losing himself in the bag of fast food as he rifled through it. He had dark features,

Greek eyebrows, and olive skin. His beard was a manicured five o'clock shadow that accentuated his strong jawline. He was short and athletic, though much to Steph's chagrin, he wore shapeless clothing that made him look like he played poker for a living. His dingy blue jeans had food stains from using them as makeshift paper towels, and his large, unbuttoned flannel was draped over a concert t-shirt for a band that Steph thought was too loud. He worked in commercial advertising, but for a company that used words like "alternative" and "edgy" to describe itself, so it gave Shawn great confidence and even greater entitlement.

"Here you go," he said, offering Steph a breakfast sandwich.

"I can't eat that."

"Yeah, you can. They're doing a new thing with gluten-free buns. It's like, half their menu now. You're good to go."

"It's not the gluten that's the problem."

"Your doctor told you that you were allergic."

"No, he said I'm allergic to dairy. I'm trying to avoid gluten."

"Fuck. Right," he said, lowering the sandwich. "Well... is it okay if I?..."

"Go ahead. I already had a bar. I figured you'd screw up."

"Normawwee, I'd be offenned," he said through a full mouth of egg McMuffin. "But I'm reeawwy hunnree." She cringed at his mouthful of food, which he saw and swallowed to appease her. "I ordered off the dollar menu, but I swear they're making these things smaller."

They sat in silence with the occasional smacking of Shawn's maw.

"Sorry. I've been so hungry since I stopped smoking," said Shawn.

"You quit smoking?"

"M'yeah," he said, taking a bite.

"How long?"

"Like... three or four days," he said, McMuffin falling from his lips.

"I'd hardly call that 'quitting.'"

"I'm on the patch. It's a process."

"I was kind of hoping you'd bring Levi with you. Where is he?"

"At my mom's," he said. "Don't worry about him, he's being spoiled. They just got satellite. He's having a field day."

"Maybe you should have brought him by."

"I wanted to see your brother first. Just to make sure it was okay."

"'Okay?' Shawn, he fell off his bike. He wasn't decapitated."

"He was hit by a car, hun. I didn't want to walk into this blind and see the guy missing an eye, caked in blood. This shit can be pretty jarring, you know?"

"I know."

Shawn felt immediate regret. He thought of something to say but decided to let his mistake slip into the past and eat his sandwich. They stared at Josh for a moment, lying in his bed, bruised but breathing.

He was right, Steph thought. It was jarring. It was haunting. Every time she looked at him, it was a violent surprise, reminding her of the reality and the stakes. Even when her eyes drifted from him, searching for comfort of any form, he was there. She scoured the recesses of her mind, grasping at wistful memories, or clutching to future errands that would demand her attention, only to be virulently jolted back to this room. Even when she went home to shower, to eat, to sleep, it was always there, waiting for her. And when she came back to him in the morning, it was here to welcome her with open arms.

"How's Martin's place?" she asked.

"Fine. He has me staying in his office on an air mattress. It's actually not that bad."

"Mhm."

"Martin is a different story, though. Since the divorce, he has become such a weird dude. Thank god I'm hardly ever there; I've been trying to stay at work as late as I can. But every time I come home, or I mean to his place..." He stopped, letting his mistake linger as if to guilt her.

"Yes? You were saying?" she said, sensing his tactic.

"He just got a virtual reality headset. It's one of the ones that you can hook up to your PlayStation, and it has these immersive headphones. He also attached these two, little sensors to the corners of the room so it can track your movement. I came home, and he pushed the couch and coffee table to the walls to make more room. He's made the entire living room into a VR court. It's maddening. He's always on it, and he looks like a fucking idiot. He shouts constantly because he can't hear himself. He's obsessed with these military games, so he says shit like, 'I'm taking fire over here!' or 'He's got a grenade!' He's up all hours of the night. I can't fucking stand it, man. It's going to give me PTSD, but a really lame version."

She laughed, which he enjoyed. He was fishing for it all along, and he got it. She could feel herself warming to him, pulled into his radiant charm. It felt familiar, and a respite from the reminder that persisted beneath everything. But she couldn't let him win. She pulled back, fortifying her initial position.

"And how are you and Courtney?"

Shawn scowled, his gaze moving to the linoleum floor, shaking his head.

"Come on, hun. You know there's nothing there."

"I don't know anything, apparently."

"It was just texting. We didn't fuck."

"In a way you did. Emotionally, you did."

"What?"

"Your mind's fucked."

"What?" He laughed at her absurdity.

"I don't need to explain myself. Don't gaslight me, Shawn. You were lying. Simple as that."

Shawn stood, pacing as if he were about to rant. Instead, he just huffed and leaned against the alabaster hospital walls, the same way her father had, his hands stabbing into his pockets with a petulant groan. Steph watched as he recalculated.

"Steph. I want to come home. Why are you doing this?"

It was her turn to laugh at his absurdity.

"I don't know. I guess I'm just crazy," she said, mocking him with a rolling finger to her temple.

"I just want things to be normal," he said. "It was harmless texting. Why is this impossible for you to overcome? Why can't you get over this?"

"Of course, you make it my problem. It's always me acting like a bitch or overreacting. It never occurs to you that you could be the one who fucked up."

"How was it flirting, hun? Just answer me that."

"We've been over this. Are you seriously this obtuse?"

"Explain it to me. How is that flirting?"

"It's flirting because that's how you flirt. You joke. You use humor, and that's what those texts were. They were jokes."

"That's not true. That's not how I flirt."

"It is. That's how you flirted with me."

"No. I mean, yes joking is part of it, but it's entirely different. I joke in general, so that's like saying I'm flirting with everyone."

"Well..." she said, implying something.

"I touch. That's how I flirt. Remember? Like when we met at Carrie's party, and we were hanging out in the kitchen? I flirted with you."

"Yeah, exactly. You joked with me."

"But I also touched your hand on the kitchen counter. You don't remember?"

She nodded as if she did, but she didn't.

"And then, if you remember, I touched your shoulder. After every time I made you laugh. It was friendly but intimate. Like this..."

He sauntered towards her, a big, dumb grin on his face, traveling backward through time to a moment when they were unfamiliar with one another.

"Hi. I'm Shawn. I gotta say, I'm a little surprised you're friends with Carrie. She usually only hangs out with women who are visibly vegan. When I walked in and saw you, the only woman who was not wearing a hemp scarf, I was confused but also immediately drawn to you."

As Steph gave a tiny chuckle, remembering the dumb line he had used, she felt his hand land on her shoulder. She looked up, staring into his coffee-colored eyes. She let it rest there for a moment, allowing things to be normal, then shrugged it off. Shawn frowned and retreated to his post against the wall. They were both painfully back in the present.

"If you want me to bring the boy by, I'll do it. I just know how much he loves Josh, and I was kind of hoping this would be a quick thing. But now that I'm seeing him, I'm kinda glad I didn't bring him."

"I get it," she said. "It could be scarring, but maybe it'd be good for him. Maybe this would be a good learning experience. I don't know..."

She didn't succumb to doubt very often, and it was a surprise to even her that she was becoming diffident. She wavered and retreated into herself.

"Part of me just needs to see him," she said. "The selfish part. I know that sounds terrible, but I think I need to see Levi."

"Well, why don't we meet up at home?"

"I'm rarely there. I've only left for two hours, so far. I can't tear myself away, Shawn. Not right now."

"How long are you going to do this, hun?"

"I don't know. As long as it takes. I've already talked to work, and they're going to allow me to work from home, or I mean, I can work from here. The Wi-Fi is really good, the university is going to give me a computer. I can do that for two weeks, then I can take vacation time; I have loads saved up. If I have to dive into my sick time... I'll cross that bridge when I come to it."

She was expecting push-back from him, her provocative tone fishing for a reaction. But he only listened, his forehead wrinkled and his eyes empathetic.

"Look, I know I fucked up the breakfast sandwich situation," he said. "But if you need me to pick up some stuff from work or from home, I'll gladly bring it by."

"Actually, yeah. Can you go by work and pick up that computer? Also, a few things from my desk; I'll text you what, exactly."

"Great. Just let the university know I'm coming by. I don't want to get stopped by security because I was exiting the building with a computer that I thought was yours, and then say something dumb like, 'My wife told me I could have it.'"

She gave a light laugh but didn't quash this one. She let him have his victory.

"I'll bring Levi next week," he said. "He's getting excited for Halloween, and he's kind of bogged down with soccer this week."

"Oh no, that's right. I'm missing the tournament."

"He understands. You're not missing much, just a bunch of running around. It's just a herd of over-sugared children, clustering around a soccer ball for two hours."

"Yeah. That's what I love about it," she said, wistful. But again, she was pulled back to her brother in his bed. "I can't explain why, but I can't leave him. It's like I'm being held captive. Even when I leave, I'm still here."

"I'll bring the boy by. It'll be good for both of you. He won't stop talking about you."

Shawn shuffled over to Josh, finally ready to get a closer look. He inspected the wounds on his face. His bruises, the cuts, the coloring of his skin. It was like examining a globe, the various continents, and landscapes of texture. Scabs, discoloration, lacerations. Shawn wrestled with his rising panic.

"I loved-" he stopped himself. "I love this guy."

Steph frowned at his past tense but decided to let it go. He was no Raina.

"I was terrified of him once," he said. "Which is hilarious because he's the least terrifying person you'd ever meet. So friendly, so funny, so willing to be stupid. But that's not what I was expecting. When we first started dating, the way you talked about him, you made him sound like this intellectual, uber-talented genius. Your brother, the software engineer.

Your admiration was so obvious, you oozed adulation for him. It was so fucking intense and intimidating. I felt like I had to stack up like you were always comparing me to him. So when you told me that we were finally going to meet, I was nervous as fuck. I did a ton of research. Did you know that? I researched the hell out of his job. I found out specifically what he did, what kind of stuff he was working on. I memorized a bunch of nonsense words, or at least they were nonsense to me. Do you remember what we did?"

"No," said Steph. "Wasn't it, like, mini-golf or something?"

"We went bowling," he said. "And of course, he's nothing like I expect. Self-effacing, warm, clumsy. Funny as fuck. The least arrogant dude I've ever met. And more importantly, he didn't want to talk about work at all. I threw out one of my memorized terms, and he shrugged it off like he didn't give a shit. And then, I never told you this, but when you were bowling he leaned over to me and asked, 'So how serious is it? Are you guys sleeping together?' And I was stunned. But then he just started busting up laughing. So I laughed too until he leaned back in and said, 'But seriously if you ever hurt her, I'll kill you.' So I was frozen again, but he just busted up again. I couldn't get a read on the guy. It was maddening."

"Oh my god, that's so unlike him," she said, enthused to have learned something she didn't know about her brother.

"And on top of it all, he was the worst bowler I'd ever seen," said Shawn. "I was winning because I was trying, but Josh didn't give a shit. He enjoyed how terrible he was. He'd throw gutter-balls and then pump his fist like he was on his way to bowling a three hundred. When we were finished, they had karaoke in the bar area, and Josh insisted that we go. Karaoke in a bowling alley, man. It was so depressing.

"I slightly remember," said Steph. "No one was good, and there were only like, two dozen people. We sat in that booth in the back."

"Yes! And I kept making fun of the singers, but Josh kept cheering them on. Then that girl got up, the real introverted one. You remember her?"

"I can't say that I do," said Steph, marveling at the details of the story he possessed.

"She was super shy," he said. "She looked like she was part bird, she was so small. And the song she chose came on, and it was 'Bad Mama Jama' by Carl Carlton. Which was hilarious because here's this tiny, shy woman, probably a preschool teacher who was just trying to have a little fun, and she picked a song that was so confident and fucking boister-ous. Just the opposite of her. If you're not a confident person, why would you pick the most confident song of all time? And everyone in the bar starts dying laughing as this mousy girl whispers her way through it. But then, I looked for Josh, and I realized he wasn't there. Then I heard people cheering. I looked, and he was next to the stage, dancing. He danced like a total dork, just like he bowled. But it was completely without irony. It was so well-intentioned and in full support of the singer. It was beautiful."

Steph closed her eyes, remembering. She tried to revisit the moment. She could almost feel that bar, that room. The corny lights that moved along the walls, illuminating a disco ball. The small screens spread throughout, all displaying the yellow lettering of the lyrics so the bar patrons could follow along. The smell of shoe polish and dried beer. She could almost hear the song.

She did hear the song. It was unmistakable. She opened her eyes to find Shawn dancing to it. His phone rested on Josh's chest, blasting the song as loud as its tiny speakers would permit. Shawn writhed and wiggled in the middle of the room, replicating Josh's cheesy dancing.

"They say music is good for brain function."

Steph laughed as Shawn put on a display of outdated dance maneuvers: the boo-ga-loo, the shopping cart, the lawn-mower, the Travolta finger guns from *Grease*. It was a revolving door of repugnant, disco-era pomp, but it was done with flamboyant conviction.

Her laughter ceased, abruptly. Shawn was confused why she had decided to suppress it. Steph's face was red as she stared at the doorway. Shawn turned to see a nurse standing behind him. He scrambled for an excuse.

"Joints got stiff on me," he said. "All this sitting around and whatnot. Trying to get up and get moving, what with fall upon us, you don't want them to go rigid. You see that all the time in your profession, I'm sure."

The nurse ignored him as she crossed to Josh's chart. She examined the various machinery, making notes regarding his pulse and blood pressure. Shawn, meanwhile, threw Steph a look, mouthing, "Why didn't you tell me?" She shrugged, impudently.

The song kept playing, serving as the soundtrack to the nurse's note-taking. Shawn sauntered over to his phone. But before he shut it off, he turned to the nurse.

"I don't know if it says so on your chart, but this guy is one hell of a dancer. Terrible bowler, but one hell of a dancer."

CHAPTER NINE

THE PULSATING BEAT OF A FUNKY, DISCO JAM THUMPED through the walls of the Sears Tower office as Josh sauntered through the aisles of cubicles. His swaying strut was similar that famous '70s actor, the one who at the end of that one movie had decided he had no choice but to walk the streets of New York with flamboyant confidence. Josh's verve was on full display, having been stoked by his factious acolytes who were offering up their undivided attention. His coworkers had become a perennial audience, one whom incessantly stood, gawking with worship. They fawned over every little thing he did, and Josh absorbed the affection, soaking in all he could.

He wasn't sure how long he had been here; the days ran together like the lazy river of a water park, continually flowing in an endless circulation that guided him through passing memories. They lazily drifted past, Josh watching them, only to see them return to him again as no day was punctuated with an end, just the same familiar faces that fomented the same fading memories. He felt as if he had been here for eternity, but also as if he had just walked through the door. The warm milieu of acquaintances was there to greet him and refused to wane or threaten to recede.

"There he is!" cheered Greg Banks, the camp counselor. "The man with the cleanest bunk in camp!"

"You know it, partner!" said Josh. "She just needed a bit of elbow grease."

Pat Perlola, the game show host, slapped an overly manicured hand on Josh's shoulder.

"You've been crushing it, fella. You're the best contestant we've had in decades."

"Well... Is that your final answer?"

Josh couldn't remember where he knew that line from. He knew it didn't belong to Pat Pelola, but nonetheless, it landed with a crushing blow, causing raucous laughter throughout the office. Lou Featherman, the news anchor, pointed from across the room.

"This Just In: Josh is amazing!"

"Breaking News: I'm aware, Lou!"

Laughter. Lots of it. Sonorous knee-slapping and guttural approval as boisterous mirth inflated the office floor. The Italian Chef came running up to Josh. He clung to his side, tears streaming down his face.

"I just-a want to-a thank you, Josh. The base-a-ball metaphor that you-a used-a helped me double my product-a-tivity. You are-a beautiful man! You are my-a hero! Bellissimo!"

"No," Josh stopped. He turned to the dozens of smiling faces, all lovingly fixed on him. "You guys are. You guys are the champions. Because without you, this whole thing wouldn't work. And we wouldn't be the best at whatever it that we do. So give yourselves a hand."

Josh applauded, encouraging everyone to clap along.

They joined, most of them tearful, as they basked in the glow of Josh.

"Nice goin', Joshy," said Andy, appearing at his side and elbowing him sharply. "You've become a regular celebrity around here."

"There he is!" boomed Big Boy Bear as he lumbered towards him. "I know what you could use, Josh."

He enveloped Josh in a gentle hug, pressing him into the soft fabric of his stuffed belly. Josh closed his eyes, allowing the sweet fragrance of the detergent from his childhood to seep into his nostrils. It sparked the synapsis of his brain, stirring memories of towels, sheets, pajamas, and sweaters, all washed with the same softener and detergent. Big Boy Bear was warm and smelled of comfort.

"Thanks for the hug, Big Boy."

"No, Josh. Thank you. You've made a big impact here."

"No bigger than the impact that the Italian Chef's ravioli has made on my waistline!"

As if the heavens themselves had split, the office exploded with atmosphere-shattering laughter. It was so exaggerated, so over-the-top, that Josh had dropped to the floor out of fear for his life. He thought a bomb had hit the city. But the laughter sustained like the exultant throng of a Madison Square Garden audience. The violent quake rippled through every member of Josh's past, every being seized with spasmed screaming. Brandon Bass buckled, his face crimson as he gasped for air. Leia Foth clutched her side, her abdomen tightening as if it were a giant's hand, crushing her ribs like a pack of toothpicks. Pat Perlola convulsed on the ground, enraptured within a savage clonic, writhing and contorting as if God were toying with him. Mr. Weeks, who was in his office and couldn't possibly have heard the joke, barrel-rolled out of his office and onto the carpet with the gusto a runaway circus clown. He sustained a high-pitch scream, his eyes bulging from his skull, tongue curled, veins popping from his neck, seemingly in terrible pain. He leaped to his feet, still scream-laughing, and ran around the office kicking over computers and turning over desks. Papers flew into the air. A small fire was started in a wastepaper basket by a chuckling employee. Office supplies were thrown as if they were cafeteria food. Anarchic mirth had infected Josh's coworkers, causing an outbreak of deranged madness.

Josh stood, frozen and confused, as he watched the chaos ensue. It was deeply unsettling, so much so that he had already forgotten what joke had prompted it all.

"Wanna get a drink?" asked Andy, ignoring the societal breakdown occurring around them.

"You can drink?" asked Josh.

"Ha! Funny, Joshy. Your funniest joke yet. Come on."

Andy started for the elevators, maneuvering around Tyler Willard, the trumpet player from Josh's band class, as Tyler brandished his horn, swinging it around wildly, bashing it into the screens of computers. He blew into the brass with warped notes, the horn bent and almost unplayable.

"Is it okay to leave them like this?" Josh asked. But Andy was already in the elevators, beckoning him with a curled finger.

They walked the streets of familiar faces and smiles. Josh tried to keep up with Andy, while also politely nodding to every familiar face.

"Where are we going?" asked Josh.

"Our favorite bar. The Gingerman."

"The Gingerman," said Josh with wistful recollection. "I love that place. Free pool, killer jukebox."

"We're meeting some people there. Wait til you see," said Andy, a rascally grin creeping across his face.

They reached a flooded intersection, people crammed together as they wiggled to cross.

"Hurry up, let's make the light," said Andy as he dashed into the crowd, scudding toward the corner. But Josh, being the much larger person, had a difficult time weaving through the crowd. Roves of smiling faces brushed past, their shoulders tightly pressed to his. School teachers and family friends smiled as they squeezed by. The current of nostalgic citizens was forceful, and Josh struggled to squeeze his way upstream.

The unfamiliar face. The face of the woman Josh had seen from across the street. The one he did not recognize. She brushed past him, locking eyes. But as soon as she appeared, she had vanished into the crowd. The tide had now changed as the sea of people reversed, pushing Josh in the original direction he had intended, which was away from the direction that the mysterious woman had disappeared into.

He made a snap decision and fought his way upstream towards her. It was harder than before, the crowd becoming dense as if it had ossified into a fortified onslaught. Her face appeared sporadically, frenetically manifesting on the shoulders of different people. As soon as he'd find her, her visage would vanish and appear in another place, on another set of shoulders. She was a transmission that couldn't quite stabilize. Her image leaped from being to being, hopping through the crowd with the ease of a frog on lily pads. Josh decided to lower himself to the pavement, slumped in a crouch, elbowing the shambling legs as he moved his way through the tumultuous sea of knees and shuffling shoes. He elbowed between kicking legs, his anxiety slightly assuaged for the time being as there was an absence of faces. He saw the bottom of her black trench coat wafting as it floated through the crowd. It took a hard left, eschewing the cloistered hysteria. He followed and saw her legs finally break free. They stood in an alley, totemic and alone. Her pointy heels slowly turned, awaiting his arrival.

Josh came tumbling out of the crowd, rolling onto the palms of his hands. They had somehow made it to a bare city alley. Still slumped over his hands, he lifted his gaze to see the face of the woman he did not know. She wore a balanced expression, neither smiling nor scowling. Josh climbed to his feet.

"Hello, Joshua."

"Hello..."

"Come with me."

"Who are you?"

"That doesn't matter. Now is the time. Come with me."

"I'm not so sure I should..."

"And why is that?" she asked with slight exasperation.

"Andy warned me about you."

She scoffed.

"Why don't you come with me and we can talk about him and this place on our way?"

"On our way where?"

"You needn't worry about that. I'll explain on the way."

"I'm sorry, but I don't think I can."

"This place is temporary, Joshua. It believes that it knows you, but you don't know what it's capable of. You need to come with me."

Josh was disturbed by her threatening tone. Her words were phlegmatic and honest, or at least it seemed. He couldn't tell. She was very still, an enigmatic shadow of a person who had the confidence to stand upright without so much of a lean to one hip.

"Who are you?"

"You don't have long."

She offered her hand over the chasm between them. Josh

observed it, feeling as if he should grasp it. A prosperous hand, or a limb of doom, Josh was unsure. Instead, he parried with a joke.

"I don't know, my momma always told me not to go anywhere with strangers!"

Her galvanized eyes stayed grappling with his.

"Are you sure?"

"Well, Andy and I were going to go grab a drink. Why don't you come?"

"You're going to regret that, Joshua," she said.

"Why?"

"Maybe stop asking so many questions," she said, curtly. Her firm composure had melted. He could see that she was annoyed.

"I'm sorry," said Josh. "I just don't know you."

"We'll have our chances. But it's going to get harder. Just try to hang on, okay?"

"Sure. Okay."

The ground quaked, tremulous as it reverberated like a rolling drum. The sound of cracking stone and chattering brick rumbled through the alleyway. Splintering wood and fracturing glass shot through the atmosphere as the earthquake intensified.

"Oh god, what is that?" said Josh as he fell to his knees.

The buildings overhead undulated and waved. Terror and raging fantods boiled in his stomach as he hunkered down, waiting for the calamity to pass. He looked up to see the Sears Tower, the beloved building and his place of work, snaking through the air like a black mamba slithering in the sky.

"What is happening?" he cried, but it fell on deaf ears as the woman had disappeared.

With a gradual peter, the quaking finally ceased. Josh lay

on the pavement of the alley, staring at the sky. His heart thumped, his head ached, and his muscles were sore. He felt as if he'd been kicked in the face, his jaw busted, his noes bruised and bloodied.

There was silence until there wasn't. A hushed scratching. While it didn't shake the ground as the quake had, a rumbling pulsated through the pavement. The sound climbed Josh's hands like the marching of a thousand tiny men. He heard a high-pitched whistle in the distance intensifying as it drew closer. Josh searched for the source of the rumbling scream. Still seated on the ground, he turned to face the end of the alley.

A black void rustled towards him, a thousand moving parts as it clamored its way through the buildings. It was a dark wave, bursting up the brick walls, over and underneath dumpsters. The water bombarded and enveloped everything in its path. As the water came closer, Josh could see that it was not water. It was rats.

The vermin stampeded, scurrying for their lives. There were thousands. Josh hurried, scrambling to his feet, but he was too late. He was engulfed and slammed onto his back, his head smashing into the pavement. The sky disappeared as the flood of fur, tails, teeth, and claws all scurried over him. He shook and fought, convulsing. They were running beyond him, feverishly rushing to an unnamed higher ground. They were seeking asylum. Rabid animals had been released upon a world that despised them, but they now made it known that they, along with the likes of them, were members of its population.

CHAPTER TEN

JOSH WRITHED IN HIS HOSPITAL BED. HE SHOOK violently, tremoring and convulsing as his teeth chattered and his jaw nibbled at nothing. "Beeps" and "dings" and "clicks" went off from the surrounding machines like demonic slot machines. Steph stared at her brother as he morphed from peaceful sleeper to a trembling body seized by a vengeful clonic. It was a possession. Ghoulish terror had gripped his body and rattled it with fury. A deity had lashed out at him in anger, demanding that he suffer for the sins committed by generations of unknown miscreants. Steph knew this was a virulent act of holiness. Or unholiness. Had he done something to deserve this? Had she?

"Help! Someone!" was all she could cry.

Lisa stood with her knees in a slight bend, pinned against the wall, but appearing ready to spring into action. However, this was not the case. Each tendon had frozen in place. Her hands were outstretched, attempting to convince whoever would listen that they could be of use. They tremored with her boy, appearing to any spectator to be the torturous instruments causing her son's fit. She looked to be manipulating the chaos like a puppeteer.

Rich had run to retrieve a nurse. He returned with several. No one could really say how many due to the nurse's frenzied movements which caused them to appear out of focus; they were other-worldly beings of swift-moving light. Their presence was not a relief. To Steph, Lisa, and Rich, they were many versions of the same person, drifting around the room as blurs of jewel-toned scrubs. They were beings comprised of nervous systems, brainless as they merely reacted to the events around them. The colors of their garments were boundless as they radiated throughout the room, bleeding into one another, orbiting the shaking body.

"Fixed pupils," one of them said. "Right and left."

"Here we go, we're moving him," said another. "Try to hang on, Josh." Steph felt comforted for a brief moment by the tender use of his name.

The sounds from the many machines had conflated into a high-pitched scream, which had filled Steph's ears and replaced any and all sound. It was the sound of confusion, pain, and incapability.

Medical terminology flew around the room, between the swirling beings with unceremonious rote.

"He's hemorrhaging."

"It might be a burst blood vessel."

"He's bleeding. Get Doctor Kaspin."

They were engulfed by the high-pitched tocsin as laconic, hospital argot was muttered underwater.

"Where are you moving him?" Lisa managed to ask.

"Surgery," said a beam of light.

"Surgery?"

Doctor Kaspin entered, flummoxed but focused. He surveyed the machinery, the flashing screens, the angry

sounds. He deciphered the language, and his muscles tight-
ened. Terse language was thrown to the beings with an
authoritative tone. Josh's bed was wheeled out.

Doctor Kaspin approached Lisa with great care.

"He's bleeding. Which is putting tremendous pressure on
the parietal lobe. He's going into surgery, and we're going to
do everything we can to stop it before there's any permanent
damage to the longitudinal fissure. If we don't act now, parts
of the brain will begin to die off."

Maybe Lisa said something. Maybe Rich did. Steph
knew for certain that she did not. Doctor Kaspin was gone,
following the hospital bed as it tore through the hallway.
Steph marveled at the way it ripped through space, like a
speed boat slicing through placid water, leaving a wake of
horror behind it. A hand touched her shoulder.

"I'll have someone show you exactly where we'll be
taking him. It's going to be a few hours. Please don't hesitate
to let someone know if there's anything else you need. Try to
hang on."

The numbness of a natural disaster. Bewilderment
bounced from person to person as each family member
turned to one another for answers. The air stiffened,
congealing into a robust thickness that kept each person in
place, solidifying their positions as statues in a diorama of
anguish. It was the epiphany of an acknowledgment towards
the possibility of mightier powers, a tacit tip of the hat that
nothing was within anyone's control. The unreasoned and
unreasonable had risen to rear its unknown countenance to
remind those who had forgotten, that it had always been and
will always be. It had a larger hand in this, and all matters
than any of the ignorant masses had convinced themselves. It
was after blood and bone. Its unrelenting rapaciousness
swelled, enveloping Steph's past, present, and future. She felt

foolish for believing she could convince herself of any reality other than the one she was firmly planted in at this very moment. This was always coming.

She stared at the ceiling where she found a water stain forming like a cloud in the sky. What all had it seen? Why was this the first time she had noticed it? It had been present for every step of this ensuing drama, existing before Steph had known. It felt sentient as if it knew every outcome. She felt that she owed it something: penance, respect, supplication. She needed to afford it power, then ask for it to use that power to restore her hope. She desperately needed it to care for her.

The hand of the nurse returned. And another. Steph was enveloped in a hug, brittle hands clinging to her and drawing her in. But it was not the nurse, it was her mother. As Steph stared at the formidable watermark, she gave her mother the comfort she prayed would soon come to her.

CHAPTER ELEVEN

A YOUNG HAND GRABBED FOR JOSH, CLUTCHING TO HIS collar, pulling him from the ground and out of the alley. He turned to see the worried face of his twelve-year-old best friend.

"Hey, bud. Lost you for a minute. You okay?"

Josh checked himself over, surprised to find himself intact.

"Yeah, I guess. Holy hell, did you feel that?"

"Feel what?"

"The earthquake... and did you see all those rats? Where the hell did they come from?"

"Ha! You sound like you're losing your shit, Joshy. Now stop messin' around, we gotta meet some people."

"What about the lady?"

"What lady?"

Josh looked around, searching for the woman in black, but she was gone.

"There was a woman. She appeared in the crowd, she

was wearing all black. She led me here to the alley. She wanted me to come with her."

"What did I tell you about her, Joshy? I told you to keep away. She's no good. She's super weird. A total creep. Just hang with me, man."

Andy led Josh back into the busy street of bustling citizens; the megacity denizens hurried over the sidewalks and roads at an intense pace. The chaotic swirl was devoid of a fixed direction and swept Josh up, throwing him every which way. This was a far bumpier ride than the rush of city patrons whom Josh had been clustered with before. This was a feverish tide, frenetic and brutish. They jostled him back and forth with hard elbows and sharp shoulders. The city as a whole was a hurried collection of peevish individuals, rudely squeezing their way past one another, muttering low-tones of querulous whispers that simmered beneath every movement as everyone seemed to be in everyone's way. Viperish shouts of frustration were hissed into the ether as each individual had become enraged by every other individual's chelonian pace.

Andy slipped through the crowd as Josh did his best to follow closely behind. He felt that something had changed within him, something of immense profundity. Darkness had swelled at the pit of his stomach, ballooning with dread and torpid weariness. There was a reverberation of doubt and fear: that which was once promising and fruitful had wizened and withered into a rotten forgone conclusion. It was emulous of the dread he felt in the quintessential "big test nightmare"; the one where he had somehow forgotten to study for the exam and showed up to class nude. The fetid miasma of encroaching failure had unleashed rancorous nausea, causing a rise of roiling consternation that ignited his throat and gave him a pounding headache. The fantods in his gut had manifested visually as the city seemed in disrepair. The buildings that were once shining beacons of prodigious beauty had decayed into vestigial versions of their aged selves.

The Chicago Tribune Building was covered in a sporing mold, looking weather-beaten and lugubrious. Streaks of mud-stained ice had melted into rivulets of sludge that gave it the decoration of feces colored pinstripes. The beleaguered building reflected the now opaque, portentous overcast that had seized upon the sky and submerged the city. The Lincoln Memorial was missing bricks of marble, seemingly under haphazard renovation. As Josh rode the surge of crowd past, he peered inside to find the crestfallen Lincoln sitting on his throne without his head; it sat firmly in his lap, its listless eyes gazing into nothingness.

The bumping intensified. Shoulders slammed into his, elbows stabbing into his ribs and chest, pointed hips bounced him from body to body. People fought for positioning, struggling with one another as they did everything they could to gain any semblance of advantage. The crowd stopped at a light, waiting. The space around Josh, what little belonged to him, evaporated as citizens inched closer. The pressure built like rising steam. The heat intensified as the bodies pressed into Josh's. Pressure, heat, squeezing, smothering. The coats of known strangers rose to Josh's face, warming the air around him into an unbreathable haze. He was in a vice that gripped with sedulous force and malevolent intentions as it sought to grind his ribs into fractured kindling.

There was a crack of daylight. Josh slipped through, achieving fresh air for the first time in what felt like an eternity. He crossed the street to an open corner inhabited by no one except for a waiting Andy.

"What was that all about?" asked Josh. "Why is everyone so pushy?"

"Lunchtime, man. Everyone has someplace to go, and we're no exception. Come on, dude."

Acrid smoke filled Josh's nostrils. It was the recognizable singeing of fabric and burnt cotton, but he didn't know where it was coming from. It put him on primal alarm. He searched around him, seeking its source. His gaze finally rested on Andy who stood as he had before except with a small flame perched on his shoulder like a canary. It grew and grew as Josh struggled to leap into action.

"Andy."

"What's up, bud?" he said, oblivious to the growing flame.

"The fire."

Josh yelped, his fear bubbling from the back of his throat. He thought of nothing to do but to envelop Andy in a hug, squelching the flames. He smothered him into his chest, holding him close. Andy felt hot and wreaked of burnt plastic. There was an inorganic smell of fabrics and textures whose purpose was never to be welded together. As Josh pulled away, he saw that Andy's clothes were sprinkled with torched blotches, as if he had attempted suicide with a Bic lighter and gave up. His skin was unblemished, although, it had grown a shade pinker.

"Woah," said Andy. "Close one. Nice save, Joshy."

"I shouldn't have moved. I should have stayed. I could've done something."

"Why would you say that? That was beyond your control, man."

"Maybe if I would have fought harder, convinced my parents that we had to stay?"

"I appreciate the sentiment, but we have places to be, dude."

Andy carried on, ambivalent to the traumatic events of the past and present. They went to cross the street, and Josh saw Big Boy Bear standing on the opposing corner.

"Hey, Big Boy!" Josh called to him.

But the stuffed bear only returned a perfunctory wave. He paced, lumbering back and forth, lost in thought. As they grew closer, Josh made out Big Boy's furrowed brow. He was sullied, dirty. His once clean coat was now a spavined hide with stains and grey bruising. There were areas of his tawdry stitching that had come undone, the tufts of fluffy white protruding like tiny smokestacks. He wore a baleful expression, shaking his head in exasperation.

"That mother fucking cocksucker has some mother fucking nerve," said Big Boy Bear.

Josh saw that the irritable bear was now smoking, a cigarette sitting between his rotund fingers. He puffed on it wildly, gesturing with fledged experience. "Mr. Weeks can suck a fat fucking dick."

"What happened, Big Boy?" asked Josh.

"Get this. Weeks' wife comes into work today, she brought him lunch or whatever. So I'm in the break room, and this bitch is sitting there microwaving something. And I'm waiting there, planning on heating up a cup of fuckin noodles. All of a sudden she bends over, grabbing something from under the sink. And you've seen her. I mean, the ass on this chick. And she's got this itty-bitty skirt on her. So I check her out, and she must have caught me out of the corner of her eye. She spins around and she fuckin glares at me! It's like, why the fuck are you wearing the skirt then?! So, she runs to Weeks and tells him that I fuckin hit on her. I didn't say one fuckin word, man! Not one. So he's chewin me out, and I'm like fuck you, man. I slave for that fucker. I'm on the phone, god knows how many hours, dancin and singin for this piece of shit client list who don't give a flyin fuck about me, or my mortgage, or my god damn car payment. All because your whore of a wife wants a little attention? Fuck her and fuck Weeks."

Josh stared at him in disbelief.

"Do... do you want a hug?" Josh asked.

Big Boy sucked on his cigarette with bristling acrimony, his black button eyes peering deep into Josh's fearful ones.

"No. I want a fuckin drink, Josh."

"Well, you're in luck," said Andy. "We're on our way to the Gingerman."

"Beautiful. I need some fuckin whiskey, or I'm gonna blow my fuckin brains all over the sidewalk. Fuck, I need a vacation. Or maybe I just need to get my dick wet. Either way, let's get to this fuckin bar."

Big Boy trudged ahead, his puffy, soiled legs pounding the pavement as his spine curved-over like that of an exhausted door-to-door encyclopedia salesman from the '50s. Andy strode next to him, the edges of him burnt and smoldering. They complained to one another about the hardships of the modern day lower-middle class. Josh merely listened, still shocked by the asperity that radiated from every nook and cranny of the city and his friends. He ran through the areas of his mind in search of the misstep that he must have made to incite such rancor. Why was there an air of reproach lingering about him? What had he done wrong? He was wandering through an aftermath, which must have resulted from something he had done. Josh had no idea what, but it surely must have been a blasphemous folly of his doing.

He begged for forgiveness for a forgotten act. He only wanted the arenicolous dread that festered in his stomach to cease, for his friends to quell their vengeful bitterness, and for the world to soften again. He looked towards the horizon and saw a forest just beyond the city. Canopying the large timbers were ominous clouds of whorling, black ink that were beginning to amass into hulking hills of distant storms. The system billowed like qualmish factory smoke, crawling through the sky, dragging itself towards the city. It was on its way, thought Josh. There was no stopping it.

CHAPTER TWELVE

STEPH ENTERED THE HOSPITAL CHAPEL WITH CAREFUL steps that expected disaster. Her feet tested the ground as if it were fragile ice that would break away at any moment. The ground could quake at any second, the man hanging from his cross suddenly waking to see her, someone who doesn't belong, defiantly sneaking her way into his house of worship. He would vanquish her from this earth, shattering the floor below and sending her into the void. At any moment she could be ousted as a pariah, a non-believer. She shouldn't be here.

But then again, the people who belonged here were those who had encountered severe, unprecedented misfortune. These were not worshipers, but beggars. They had come to this hospital after some unfathomable terror had unleashed itself upon their lives, sending them crawling to the nearest holy place to ask that mercy be granted. It was a temple of last resort, those who could barely recite the first four lines of their "Our Father," but who were so desperate that they were willing to strike a deal with however many gods it would take so long as they received a miracle.

Or maybe they were here to come to terms with the power of their creator, offering up their praise along with their last, meaningless demands. Other than the feeling of desperation and anguish, Steph thought it was actually a charming church. There was a half-sized organ next to a sparsely decorated alter. The windows housed intricate designs of stained glass which portrayed the mighty saints with grace and surprising elegance. The pews were a polished pine, sturdy and strong. Steph had expected the hospital chapel to be half-assed, an afterthought to those who still clung to their faith and eschewed the irony of the physical, present help who were scrambling the halls of the hospital with magic potions that could have cured every disease that had ever killed a man or created a saint. But it was not a bad-looking chapel, and much like the riskless watercolor in Josh's room, it served its purpose admirably.

There were a dozen strangers scattered throughout the pews, planted firmly in their isolation. They were either looking down with their eyes closed, or gazed at the ceiling with their eyes open. Either way, they were silent and rooted in their individual moments with their god. And there was Lisa, front and center just as Steph had suspected. She was the only visitor who stared straight ahead, her eyes empty and the muscles of her face relaxed. In her lap, her hands were neatly folded. Before she alerted her mother of her presence, Steph marveled at how little space she occupied. So small. Steph tried to pry into her mind, reading all of its contents at the moment, but she was impenetrable as usual.

"He's out of surgery," said Steph. "He's stable. They're saying his Glasgow rating is deeper, but it's hard to make estimations right now. His pupils are responsive, and his blood pressure has stabilized."

Lisa sighed, which Steph could not decipher as relief or exhaustion. Again, impossible to read.

"I am so glad I had him baptized. Just in case."

Steph rolled her eyes at this, which made the ice below her feel thinner than ever. She did not want to have a religious discussion with her pious mother, but could not bring herself to leave. Feeling the ice crack beneath her feet, she sat next to Lisa, who would not look at her.

"I miss him, and he's not even gone yet," said Lisa.

"Try to think positively, Mom."

"You don't understand. That's not your fault, but you don't understand."

Lisa looked at her hands, fiddling with her rings. They were the rings of her mother, gaudy costume jewelry that she used to buy in bulk. Lisa always thought her mother's taste in clothing, trinkets, jewelry, and knick-knacks, was ridiculous and embarrassing, but after she passed Lisa couldn't help but find these garish items to be cozy.

"He used to threaten to run away when he was upset with me," said Lisa. "The first time he did, he was four-years-old. I don't know where he got it from, it must have been something he saw on television. But it was when I threw away a cereal box, and apparently, there had been a toy inside. So, I accidentally tossed the thing, and he threw a fit and said, 'I'm running away!'"

Lisa chuckled, which eased Steph's stiffness. Her momentary frivolity was a welcomed respite from the bleak chapel atmosphere.

"And he kept doing it, which I thought was funny because it had become more and more ridiculous. The smallest thing would happen: he didn't get dessert, I asked him to go to bed, he was told to clean up his room. He would threaten to run away. It began to wear on me. And one time before school, I told him that he couldn't do something-or-other, I don't remember. But he was angry with me, and he threatened to run away. And I just snapped. So I dared him to do it. I said, 'Oh, you want to run away so bad? You want to be on your own? You think you can live without your mom? You go right ahead. Here, I'll pack your bag for you.' And I did. I packed a bag, very impetuously of course. It was his school backpack, and I put in a few clothes and some snacks. Then, I shoved it in his arms and pushed him out the door. He stood there, and I watched him. He took one step, and he started bawling. Just crying his poor little heart out. The thought of his mom not wanting him, the reality of being on his own, it crushed him. I felt awful. I let him back inside and wrapped him in my arms. But he didn't threaten to run away anymore."

She laughed, which Steph marveled at, surprised to see grief and comedy sharing a space so amicably.

"He's such a softy," said Steph.

"I scared him because sometimes that's what you have to do. But when they scare you, it's the worst."

Her mother's face turned sallow. She stopped fiddling with her rings and carefully smoothed the wrinkles out of her long skirt. She did it so gingerly, with such care that Steph felt hypnotized by the sanctimony of the scrupulous act.

"As a mother, you try to give them lessons. And you don't know what is going to stick. As you guys have grown up, you tell me stories that even I have forgotten. You kids constantly surprise me with what you've chosen to take with you. Sometimes my hardest-fought lessons are cast aside, but you manage to find the same meaning in some thoughtless act that your father or I did. But you still try. As a parent, you try to be fair, you try to guide them, and you try to protect them. But then something like this happens, and it undermines everything you've done, everything you've worked so hard for. The lessons you've bestowed. The talks. The scares. It all feels so meaningless."

Steph scrambled for a joke, hoping to rescue her mother from dipping further into her existentialism, which made her feel awful as this was surely Lisa's first venture into this deep pool where Steph was a decorated swimmer. She knew her mother had lived her life believing in justice and defined divine morality. The lesson her mother was being taught by the universe was so multi-faceted and muddy that Steph was uncertain whether or not Lisa's sanity would survive.

"Well, Josh used to tease me so much sometimes I wished he would run away." Steph forced a laugh, hoping it would infect her mother, but it fell flat. Her mother stared at her skirt, diligently smoothing out the invisible creases. It was clear that she was not, and had not, been listening. She had been talking. To Steph, maybe. To herself, possibly. To God, always. But as was her way throughout Steph's childhood, Lisa was not listening.

"He never handled death well," said Lisa. "When Shirley had hip dysplasia, and we had to put her down, he slept underneath his bed that night. When his rabbit died, he demanded that we have a funeral. We buried it in a shoebox, Rich played 'Amazing Grace' on his harmonica, and Josh said a eulogy that lasted probably twenty minutes."

"All kids have trouble with death."

"Not you."

Steph was startled by her mother's recognition. She felt less like an apparition of her mother's despondency and more like the daughter of a wallowing woman.

"No," said Lisa. "If your goldfish died you would flush it

and wave goodbye as it circled the drain. When Rita, that little alley cat we nursed back to life got hit by a car, I was worried that you'd be unable to sleep. Instead, I was up all night that night, and you slept like a baby."

Steph found this to be somewhat amusing and empowering, the thought of her having control at a young age.

"The worst came when my father died," said Lisa. "Josh had always been close to him. But his last few weeks were very dark if you remember. You were maybe too young, but he was not himself. It was hard on all of us, but much harder on Josh because he didn't understand what exactly was happening. He'd talk to my dad, who wasn't quite all there at the time, and Josh would look at me so completely confused. He couldn't remember Josh, didn't know his name. Josh had touched his hand and startled him. I tried to explain it, but it didn't make sense to him. He was only eleven, and when my dad finally passed, he ran away for real. He was missing for hours, which sounds ridiculous to say now, but back then it felt like the world was ending. He had run into those woods near the house. Some hikers found him balled up underneath a willow."

Steph remembered. She remembered because she had been lost in the shuffle that day. She was riding her bike at a neighbor's house, having only recently learned to ride without training wheels. She had been practicing her turns in their driveway, and when she took a turn too sharply, she slammed into the pavement. She had road rash on both of her shins and trickles of blood formed on her wrists. She ditched her bike and ran two houses down, back to their house. She dashed into the living room, begging her mother to tend to her wounds.

"What the hell happened?!" demanded Lisa. Her mother

never swore, except when she was angry or scared, so Steph was immediately alarmed.

"I got her. Let's go, baby," said Rich as he swooped in and took her into the bathroom. She remembered peering over his shoulder at her pacing mother.

"What's wrong?" Steph asked.

"Your brother is messing with us," he said.

When they finally reached the bathroom, her father was so absent with worry that he brutishly swabbed the scrapes with burning alcohol, while applying bandages of the wrong sizes. When her father had finished, she wandered back into the room where her mother anxiously sat, her knee bouncing as she awaited a phone call at any minute. Her nails picked at the frayed fabric on the arm of the couch from the cat, Rita, having scratched it to death. Lisa's eyes were fixed on the weather report, which reported rain on its way.

"Mom, look what happened."

"Lord in heaven, I pray that he's not out there when this rain hits."

Lisa stood and left her daughter showing her bandages to the empty cushions.

Now, they sat together in a hollow church, each begging for the attention from an almighty power that was incapable of gifting it.

"I'm so thankful that it wasn't you, Stephanie."

Steph looked to her, thrown by her odd sentiment.

"Because, honestly, had it been you, I don't know if he could have handled that. And then I would be at the risk of losing two children."

How enraging and odd, Steph thought. Steph balled her fists and gritted her teeth, coiled. But she, again, noticed her mother's frail size and sinking ennui. A wave of relief washed over Steph as she realized at that moment that her mother could not help it. She could not console. She was incapable of assisting. Steph was overcome with empathy and instead of replying with a barbarous comment, suppressed her instincts and stared straight ahead. She had let go.

"We have to try to stay positive, Mom."

"You sound like your father."

"Well, we have to," said Steph, amused to preach optimism, which was the reverse of her relationship with her husband and her brother.

"You don't understand," said Lisa.

"There's so much we don't know, Mom."

"I've seen these things, Stephanie. I was a nurse. I've seen how they shake out. I've seen patients in his situation, with his symptoms, in this very predicament. This has happened before to many, many people. There are only so few possibilities. And I've seen every outcome."

"Well. We need to stay positive."

Lisa said nothing in return. She stared at the altar, then looked at the cross. Her mother was either thinking or praying. For once, Steph hoped she was praying. A breeze brushed Steph's face which she thought was odd as they were inside. She looked for its source and found it hanging from the ceiling: a large air conditioning vent blew cold air into the room, a frigid chill swallowing her, which she welcomed because her anger towards her mother had made her sweaty. She found amusement and comfort in looking towards the heavens with the rest of the sparse congregation.

CHAPTER THIRTEEN

ANDY LED THE WAY AS BIG BOY BEAR AND JOSH followed him into The Gingerman Bar & Grill. It was a bar Josh used to frequent in college, known for its free popcorn, pool tables, various pinball machines spawned from hit movies of the '80s, and its popular weekend screenings of college football games that Josh pretended to enjoy if only for the free shots of well whiskey and talkative college girls.

But the room had an altered aura that he didn't seem to recall. What was usually such a jocular pub of lubricated mirth, pulsating with tangible possibility, was now a dismal scene of indolent drunks who stared into their glasses as if there were answers carved into the bottoms. The lights seemed dimmer than he remembered, the wood of the floor twisting and bubbling as if the planks had been left out in the rain. The scene was sparse and unpopulated, which was not what the venerable bar had been known for. He vaguely recognized the faces of some of the drunks as acquaintances from college, but the fondness he once had for them was thwarted by their doleful, empty leering. They barely acknowledged Josh's presence as he crept into the somber bar.

Josh kept moving, keeping pace with Andy, as if he stopped then a drunk would reach for him, bringing him close to regale him of the tragedy that had befallen them due to Josh's departure from their life. Josh felt responsible for their toilsome souls.

Andy led the group to a table where three old friends sat. Josh recognized them immediately and was troubled when he saw their drunken, grinning faces.

Bruno Llerna was a coworker from his day-job in college. They bussed tables together, always meeting at the end of shifts to see who collected the most tips.

"Let's compare tips!" Bruno would say, emphasizing the obvious innuendo.

They would saddle up to the bar where Mr. Neves, the homosexual owner who had a crush on Bruno, fed them bottomless beers even though they were underage. Bruno would get drunk, quickly, and lament to Josh the problems he was having at home. Bruno was tasked with taking care of his sick mother, the only one of his siblings who had stepped up to help. He'd get hammered in a hurry and become incoherent after only three beers, often telling the same story again and again, but Josh always did his best to listen. He was empathetic, knowing that although he probably wouldn't remember it, this time was important for Bruno. Josh also needed to make sure that Bruno made it home safe, untrustworthy of the intentions of Mr. Neves' bottomless beer promise.

Bruno sat at the dimly lit table in the Gingerman, the same warm smile, the same perfect dimples that drove Mr. Neves crazy.

Next to Bruno was Natalie Satterfield. Natalie and Josh

had dated for three months in his early twenties. It was a relationship that had clenched substantial negative space in his mind during what should have been a time of unwavering, youthful confidence. Natalie was diagnosed bi-polar and was malevolently manipulative. But, when the chemicals in her body allowed her to be, she could be dear and funny. Depending on the day, Josh never knew the person he was dating. When she was at her worst, she had a calculated way of making Josh feel utterly insignificant and small. At her best, she was affectionate and cuddly. She was an ever-changing creature that would take many forms according to what she wanted. Affection, help, sex, excitement. Josh and Natalie finally broke up, publicly, in a knock-down-drag-out fight at Josh's twenty-fourth birthday party at this very bar.

There she sat, slopping up her beer, staring at him. Although he tried to surmise then and there, Josh couldn't tell which Natalie was present tonight.

Lonny Bavaro was next to her, his teenage arm draped over her shoulders. Lonnie sat behind Josh during fifth period World History freshman year of high school. He was a quintessential jock, forever seeking ways to act like the cliche he thought he was supposed to be. He badgered Josh during class, incessantly nudging him to ask him to rate the hotness of so-and-so female classmate. He'd ask Josh to help him rank the size of his classmate's breasts from "Mosquito Bites" to "Most Motor Boat-able." At first, Josh felt as if he were being bullied, but it became clear that Lonnie's bravado was a hollow act that was merely designed to attract a friend. Lonny was profoundly lonely and sweet, but also undeniably annoying. While Josh still felt too uncomfortable to engage with his bombastic cohort, he gladly listened to Lonny's false masculine fables of weekend conquests, supplying him with the demanded "ooh's" and "now way's!" Most of these stories ended with the line, "And then we totally boned." Then, a fist bump or high-five with way too much aggression behind it.

Now, here he was, frozen in the state that Josh remembered him most: a fifteen-year-old boy in a decorated letterman's jacket, his sleeve festooned over the shoulders of a psychotically mercurial twenty-four-year-old. Lonny's eyes shone like an alley cat's with lascivious intentions.

"Sup, bitch," said Lonny, his lip curled as if he thought he was Elvis Presley.

"Josshh! My man, how yoo bin," said Bruno, slurring his speech terribly.

"Hey, Josh," said Natalie, completely benign. Josh was relieved. "You look like you haven't been sleeping. Your eyes have circles, and your face looks round." Ah, Josh thought, there she is.

"You mother fuckers got here just in time," said Lonny, practically yelling. "There's tons of fresh ass. Make sure to grab you some. I already got mine..." He whispered something into Natalie's ear, and she cackled, drunkenly. It was apparent that everyone at this table was well into their evening.

Big Boy made a motion towards the bartender, who immediately brought over a pitcher of cheap lager and glasses for the newcomers. Big Boy quickly poured himself a glass and guttled it down as if he had just stumbled out of an arid wasteland, the frothy booze streaming down his gulping, fuzzy neck and onto his lumpy gut. He slammed the glass down on the table as if he were making the final, winning point in a long-standing argument.

Andy poured himself a full glass, which Josh watched uncomfortably. It was an eery sight, watching a child fastidiously pour himself a glass of beer with narrowed focus so as not to fill the glass with foam.

"Can you drink, Andy?"

Andy chortled. "Can I drink?..." With that, he opened his throat and dipped the glass back. Josh watched the booze slide down his lithe larynx like the swooping drop of a roller coaster having plummeted over its tear-drop peak.

A hand clutched Josh's collar, pulling him close.

"I'm zo glad you are here, maann," said Bruno. "Itsso fucked up, dude. It has been ssoo fuckd up, man."

"Oh, I'm sorry to hear that, Bruno."

"Nah, man. My mom. She died, bro. It wreeeaally fucked me up. Like, wreeaalllyy bad."

"Oh no, Bruno. I'm so sorry. How terrible."

"It happened a while go, man. I wish I coulda talkd to yoo. But Iss cool, it juss fucked me up is all. Fuck, man."

Bruno became startled, glancing over his shoulder as if someone had said his name. He stared into an empty corner, seemingly recognizing an invisible man.

"Oh no," he said to Josh. "He's here."

Josh stared into the corner where nothing stood.

"How come you didn't tell me you knew this bitch?" asked Lonny.

"I can't believe you didn't tell him that we dated, Josh," said Natalie. "But I suppose you were always a bit aloof."

"How was he in the sack?" asked Lonny.

"Let's just say he had difficulty rising to the occasion."

Natalie laughed at her own joke, then peered out of the corners of her eyes to make sure Josh had heard. He had. Lonny burst out laughing, then crept closer to her, whispering in her ear again. After listening for a moment, she spat a mouthful of beer, laughing sloppily.

"You're so bad!" she screamed. "Stop!"

"Wait, I didn't finish! Let me finish-"

"You're up to no good!"

"Here, let me finish-"

She let him slide close again. Josh could only make out the words "pussy" and "deep," and again Natalie was spitting beer across the table, showering Josh in the frothy rain of lager and saliva. It boiled as it made contact with his skin, the devious intentions of the action souring on him.

A hand on his shoulder again. Bruno was pawing at him, trying to bring him close.

"The restaurant hazz been lousy, man. No good money anymore since you lefff, bro."

"I'm sorry to hear that, Bruno."

"I know. Annnd like, I don't know what to do. Like, if I had a lil bit to ged me back on my feet. Juss a lil bit."

"Oh."

"Yeah, I mean. Andy said you been doin really good at werk. So, you thing you could loan me a lil bit? Juss til I get back on my feet. My mom, man. It wrrreealllyy fucked me up, bro."

Big Boy lit a cigarette and puffed as he stared into space.

"Hey! No smoking!" yelled the bartender.

"How about you go fuck yourself?" said Big Boy as he turned his back on the bartender like a truculent silverback, begging him to take a shot with every advantage.

"How big is it?" asked Lonny.

"Is what?" asked Natalie.

"His dick? I always figured Josh had a huge cock."

Natalie howled with laughter. "Let's just say if it were on a fast food menu, you could find it on the kid's menu."

Lonny buckled at this sophomoric jab. A joke tailor-made for him.

"Hey, come here. Let me tell you something..." said Lonny.

He whispered into Natalie's ear, and beer squirted out her nose and spouted through her lips.

"Oh my god, you're terrible! He's sitting right there."

"So?!"

"You're a bad one! I gotta keep my eye on you."

The sound of a body stumbling through a door was Kiera falling into the bar. She came barreling in so sloppily that she immediately dropped to her knees. Josh shot up from his barstool, relieved to see her. He darted across the bar to help, but as he came close she composed herself, and Josh was alarmed by her stormy eyes. They were glassy and vacant. She was older, firmly in her thirties, and she looked dehydrated and sleepless.

"Kiera, are you okay?"

He reached for her, which spooked her. She jumped, walleyed.

"Hey, get off me, creep!"

"Keira, it's me. Josh."

As the name worked its way towards the center of her brain, her muscles finally relaxed.

"Ooohhh. Wow. I haven't seen you in forever."

"What? Keira, we've been hanging out. I saw you yesterday."

She brushed past him, a scent of menthol cigarettes and angst trailing close behind. Her hair was frayed, the skin of her face blotchy and ruptured with scabs from zits she had impetuously popped herself. The baby fat that clung to her cheeks was gone, revealing a gaunt mask. She landed at the bar and removed her signature acid-wash jean jacket, which revealed the track marks that Josh didn't want to admit he knew were there. She ordered an appletini; a drink made for a kid whose taste buds hadn't come in yet.

"Keira. Do you care to explain what's on your arms?"

She said nothing.

"Keira. Where have you been? Who have you been with? Who did this to you? Who gave you that shit?"

Again, she said nothing. Her appletini arrived, and she slurped it down. Josh grabbed her arm and twisted her towards him. Her eyes were glazed with a blanket of chalk that smothered all lucidity inside them.

"Come on, Josh. Don't be such a bummer," she said, the emotionless words fumbling out of her tranquilized lips. Josh released her, and she turned back to her drink as if the scene had just been rewound and erased.

A tap on his shoulder belonged to Andy.

"Yo, Joshy. Let me show you something."

Andy led Josh to the back of the bar where a lifeless air hockey table sat along with three pinball machines.

"The old game area," said Josh. "I can't believe it."

"Yeah, buddy. And they just got a new one. Check it out."

In the middle sat the pinball machine from his favorite childhood cartoon. It was the one about that middle-to-lower-middle-class family who were supposed to feel like they could be anyone's family. There was the controlling mother, the bumbling father, the overlooked/hard-working sister, and the goofball son. They felt so familiar to your own family but different enough to laugh at.

"I can't believe it!" said Josh. "I loved this show. You got a quarter?"

"You bet, bud."

Andy handed Josh a quarter, which he quickly inserted. The machine sprang to life with a series of clicks and flashing lights. Familiar one-liners and famous dialogue buzzed from the speakers as the characters recited prominent phrases from Josh's past. The game readied itself, delivering a silver ball to the coiled spring, its reflective surface glowing with expectation. Josh pulled back the knob, charging the firing pin, and with declarative force sent the ball careening into the machine as if he were launching a man into space, the ball bouncing through the lively mechanisms as it explored the far reaches of everything the frontier had to offer. As the ball came down, Josh rested his eager fingers on the buttons, ready to control their respective levers. But it was futile readiness as the ball split the difference, slicing directly through the middle. The machine's energy subsided, along with Josh's enthusiastic demeanor.

"What? Oh, come on."

Another ball sprang into the chamber. Josh peevishly pulled back the knob, jettisoning the ball into the machine with determined anger. But the same event occurred, the ball cutting through the middle and delivering an unceremonious conclusion. Josh was befuddled by the indignity. He launched his last ball, and he was less than surprised to witness the same action: the ball, which once held such promise, slicing through the open middle, thudding into the machine like the round pellet of an eighteenth-century soldier's ammunition into the heart of an enemy Red Coat. Josh was paralyzed and bleeding with rage. How could something he loved wrong him with such injustice?

It felt as if he were being laughed at. A known chuckling, that of a notorious playground bully, surrounding him with humiliation. But as Josh came out of his stupor, he realized that the laughter was real, and it was coming from over by the bar. It belonged to Dewey Reese.

Dewey Reese had been, not so much a bully, but more of

an aggro presence in Josh's late middle school years. Josh was mostly overlooked by Dewey until he caught Josh making an off-color joke at his expense. Josh was new in town but had managed to fall in with a small group of nerdy, sweet boys. They would gather together between periods, making fun of classmates amongst themselves. Many of them had been the subject of Dewey's gruff teasing or physical intimidation in sports or PE, so naturally, he became the subject of their waggish jabs. One boy pointed out that Dewey had already sprouted so much leg hair that he had probably been held back several grades. Another mused that Dewey's grades were so poor due to his mother and father being first cousins and not knowing it.

Josh's turn came next. Anxious and searching, he finally decided to target the boy's ratty clothes. They were dirty, smelly, and he mostly wore a small rotation of shabby blue jeans and hand-me-down skateboard tee's that had once belonged to one of his three older brothers. It just so happened that Dewey was passing by when he heard the wise-crack. He grabbed Josh by the neck and delivered a swift blow to his gut. All air left Josh's body as if every breath he had ever taken were yanked from him and every future breath would not belong to him. Dewey made a point to make Josh's life hell from then on out.

Other than being a common knuckle-dragger, Dewey also had a deep love for anything and everything mafia related. He would emphatically act-out his favorite scenes from mob movies, which usually centered around a violent explosion. He liked to act the scenes out in the hallway for what little friends, or more aptly, hostages, would politely listen. And this is what he was doing at this very moment. He stood by the bar, speaking in a nasal voice as he impersonated a famous mob actor and acted-out a famous scene in which the character had unleashed vicious punishment. The bar patrons laughed and cheered, which Dewey absorbed with a hungry smile that seemed to drip. Keira was his most attentive viewer. She blushed and chuckled, her eyelids heavy with intoxication.

Josh balled his fists into a clenched rage as one after another his short steps brought him closer and closer to the irreverent Dewey.

"So that's when the guy is like, 'Oh, I got ya money,'" Dewey imitated, his voice nasally and grating. He paused for dramatic effect, carrying himself with the showmanship of a cheap car salesman. "'I got ya money right here.' And boom! He smacks the shit out of him with the butt of his revolver! Then his crew grabs the guy, they pull him over the counter, and they just start beatin on him. Like this..." He mimed the pistol whipping while the throng of drunken onlookers lapped it up, clapping and whistling. Keira was especially entranced.

"So then what happened, Dewey?" she asked.

"They bailed outta there! The tires screeched, and the car fishtailed, and they were fuckin gone!" His hand landed on her shoulder, creeping its way up her neck to play with her hair. Their eyes flared with connection.

"But he gets it in the end," said Josh through his teeth.

Dewey stopped, seeing him for the first time.

"Heeeyyy! If it isn't Josh Husk-y! Long time no see, doofus."

"Husk-y" was a nickname coined by Dewey, which had unfortunately caught on. Josh wasn't even that corpulent at the time. Sure, he might have gained some stress weight due to the move across the country, but this was neither here nor there. Childhood teasing and nicknames demand no reason. Dewey wore an earnest grin, unfeigned in his happi-

ness to see Josh. But Josh wasn't in the mood for camaraderie.

"He gets it in the end," said Josh. "The character you're
speaking of. He gets set up and led into a hideout, thinking
he's getting made. And bam, he gets it right in the back of the
head. He was a freaking idiot."

The bar fell silent as Dewey's shoulder's tensed. No
longer was he happy to see Josh. He remembered. This was
the same little fart who teased him about his cheap clothes.
The one who made him feel inadequate for having a drunk
for a father and an absent mother who couldn't hold down a
job and refused to buy him anything other than the rags and
cotton left-overs that his brothers had almost thrown out.
Dewey's face contorted to the pugnacious look of the enemy
Josh had once known. Even though he stood in the same form
as he remembered, a fourteen-year-old boy with a unibrow
and bubbling, fresh acne, Josh was still terrified of him. Even
though he was the older of the two by over double, Josh still
felt Dewey's tight hold on a fearful section of Josh's brain that
had always been frightened of him, and both of them knew it.

"So he does, Husk-y. Yeah, he gets it in the end. But he
was a badass before that."

"Doesn't matter much if he gets a bullet in the brain."

"What are you tryinta say, Husk-y?" asked Dewey, still in
his nasal mob voice. This enraged Josh because Dewey wasn't
even Italian. What was the purpose of this masculine obsession, dammit?!

"Take your hands off Keira."

"Scuse me?"

"What's a matter, numb-nuts? Your hearing not so good?
I said Keira and I are together."

This got a hearty laugh from the crowd that had gathered;
Big Boy, Bruno, Natalie, and Lonny now standing nearby.

Dewey blushed, crimson in his embarrassment. His shoulders tensed further, climbing up his back into a bowed position like a combative brown bear. His beady eyes narrowed, the irises disappearing amidst the midnight black of his pupils. Josh watched, anxiety building. That same corner of his brain was telling him to run as it always had. But this was his world, his favorite bar, his friends, his past. Dewey was the outlier. Both stood in thick anticipation.

"You're talkin' pretty big there, Husk-y. You musta grown a pair since I last seen ya."

"Big time," said Josh. He didn't know what that meant, but it sounded right. "Hey, Dewey. You like bananas?"

"Sure."

"Then why don't you make like one and split?"

Chuckles filled the bar. Lonny especially loved the pun. Dewey fumed.

"Fat chance, Husk-y."

"You're making me sick just looking at you. We may have to start calling you 'Spewey.'"

An eruption now. Josh had won over the bar, everyone slapping their knees in unison. Keira had come back to life, shrugging off Dewey's arm and rejoining Josh's side. Her drunken arm seductively slithered over his shoulders. Josh decided to press his luck with further wordplay, taking aim at Dewey Reese's last name.

"I think we're done here. So why don't you Reese's PEACE out of here."

Genius. He had taken Dewey's last name and related it to candy. The bar laughed even harder, cementing themselves firmly on Team Josh. Dewey steamed as visible anger anchored him.

"Time to go, little guy," said Josh as he approached, plopping his hand on Dewey's shoulder, which only reached the middle of Josh's sternum. Dewey responded with a shove as if he were throwing down a gauntlet and the bar was a playground. It sent Josh back on his heels. He met Dewey's expecting gaze. Can he hit a child? It was now or never. Josh balled his left fist, cocking it back as if he were an archer preparing his bow. He sent forth the strongest punch that his physical form would permit. It wasn't pretty, by god, but it was a punch. And it landed squarely on Dewey's chin.

Dewey's face snapped to the left, absorbing the blow, but he remained standing. He returned his stare, unaffected. Josh, alarmed and riled, sent forth a slew of punches. They resembled hooks and overhands and straights and uppercuts. But they did nothing, all landing square on Dewey's peach-fuzz-covered chin like light splashes of water. Dewey sneered and walked forward as if he were stepping into a light hail storm. Josh backpedaled, the area of his brain that he had silenced only moments ago now screaming its knell of panic and doom. The laughter that once belonged to Josh and his quips had now turned against him as it targeted his pathetic display of manhood. Dewey caught Josh's final, tenuous punch, bending his wrist backward. Josh howled in pain. Dewey grabbed him by his collar and threw Josh over a table, sending him a quarter of the way across the room as if he had been gifted god-like strength. Josh skidded across the twisted floorboards of his favorite bar, rolling end-over-end in a chaotic tumble. As he rested on his back, Dewey's looming figure came into focus. Behind him, his drunken friends and acquaintances gathered with worried looks. Dewey's fist. Then his other. And again and again. They were deleterious blows of significant impact that struck at the even tempo of a healthy heartbeat. Between the strikes, Josh could hear them laughing. Keira was amongst them.

Josh relaxed, allowing the oncoming barrage to overwhelm him. It occurred to him that the beating felt very familiar to the scene from the movie that Dewey had been describing. Where the helpless shopkeep was overwhelmed by the blood-thirsty deviant and his crew. What did the shop-keep do? He strained to remember as his face reddened with flushing blood and immediate bruising.

CHAPTER FOURTEEN

LISA'S STEADY HAND GENTLY BRUSHED JOSH'S BRUISED face at a fixed, careful tempo. It was a grim image as her son looked beaten and pulpy with part of his head having been shaved for the emergency procedure. She couldn't help but stare at the intrusive wound and feel personally offended. They had pried into him and no matter their intentions, it felt fallacious and cruel. Her locked gaze was broken as a water bottle was thrust between her and her son.

"Take a sip," said Rich.

"I'm not thirsty."

"Lees. Please. You need to stay hydrated."

"I don't want any water, Rich."

"It isn't water. Well, it is, but I added an Emergen-C."

"What emergency?" she asked. "The water is under emergency?"

"No. There's Emergen-C in the bottle."

"I don't understand. Is the water no good? It doesn't look like water."

"That's how it's supposed to look!"

Steph sat by the window and quickly decoded the misun-
derstanding, but instead of clearing up the confusion, she
received it as a benison of entertainment from the gods.

"I don't know what you want me to do," said Lisa. "You're
not making any sense."

"Drink it."

"No! It looks disgusting, Rich. Why is it orange and
murky?"

"That's the Emergen-C! Look, it has lots of vitamins in it.
You haven't eaten anything, and you only took two sips of
your tea this morning. You have to stay hydrated, hun, and
this is good for your immune system. Come on, drink it."

She glared at him, but was too exhausted to take such a
ridiculous stance as "I don't need to drink fluids." She took
the bottle and helped herself to two baby sips to appease him.

"There. Satisfied?"

"What do you think? Pretty tasty, right?"

"It's the greatest non-water I've ever had, now please
throw it away."

Rich scoffed and took the bottle back to his leaned position against the wall. He muttered something like, "you try to
be nice," but it was inaudible. Steph, sitting in her usual place
in the chair by the window, returned to working on her
laptop. She was enjoying the demands of her job at this time
as they made her feel physically present, yet mentally
removed from the situation. Josh was stable, providing a
center of social gravity tantamount to a small fireplace, while
her parents puttered about the room, annoying one another.
It was cozy in a backward way.

The television filled the silence of the room with *Looney
Tunes* cartoons that Rich had turned up to such a blaring
volume that the speakers could barely house the calamity and
goofy violence. Rich chuckled along with Road Runner and

the futile efforts of Wile E. Coyote. Lisa was jealous of Steph and Rich, their ability to lose themselves in screens at this moment. Instead, she sat with glazed eyes, her focus inward as the muscles surrounding her skull felt as if they were shrinking; a brawny palm grasping to her cranium, squeezing. Her head throbbed with the dull thud of a duteous chef cleaving a chicken breast into a thin sheet. Her jaw was fused shut as the muscles in her face clenched like a crocodile's. Her brow was pinched in searing pain. She searched for the source, blaming Rich for a moment. She mustered anger towards him and his ambivalent, impudent choice to play the television so loud, but she hadn't the strength for reprobation. Wile E. hit a wall, a rock he had painted to look like a passable tunnel, but the Road Runner had been able to defy physics and pass through it. But when Wile E. had tried, he smashed into the surface.

"Uh oh! Gonna have to find another way!" Rich cackled like a child.

Lisa's head pounded; someone was at the front door and demanded to be let in.

Wile E. used a cannon in the hopes of increasing his speed, but just as the Road Runner flew by, he lit the fuse only to have the cannon blow up with him still in the barrel.

"Well, that didn't work like you thought it would!" Rich boomed.

Lisa's head thumped like a tribal drum.

Wile E. was hot on Road Runner's tail, having chased him to the edge of a cliff. But when they had reached the sharp declivity, Road Runner kept sprinting, his speed so propulsive that he was able to reach the other side. Wile E. wasn't so lucky. As he looked down and discovered the chasm below, he fell, a high-pitched whistle sounding as it took a great deal of time before he smashed into the canyon floor.

"Here's an idea: maybe next time you shouldn't look down!" Rich howled.

Her head pounded like the time she was a little girl, and she had climbed a tree with her friends and slipped and fell, hitting several branches on her way down, finally landing on the ground, a gash in the back of her skull with the thump of her heartbeat filling her ears.

"Off," she said.

"What's that, dear?" said Rich, still laughing.

"Off." It was all she could say and even that hurt.

"But this was his favorite. Ya know, I read that Chuck Jones was in a coma and his family visited him and were able to pull him out by getting him to talk like Bugs. He came out saying, 'What's up, doc?'"

"Is that true?" asked Steph, suddenly present in the room.

"I think so. Or, it may have been Elmer Fudd. But I'm pretty sure it was Bugs."

"Off."

"Fine!"

After the television was shut off, the grim silence hung about the room like morning dew. Steph tried to go back to her work, but couldn't seem to refocus. All she could think about was Bugs Bunny in a coma. His lifeless ears flopped to one side as he lay in an ACME bed. Liquidated carrots oozing through an IV and into his veins. Elmer Fudd would sit by his side, shrouded in grief. Daffy would be in the parking lot, still seated in the car, unable to gather the courage to see his frienemy in such a horrid state.

Lisa realized that without the distraction of the white noise of *Looney Tunes*, she felt as if she was being pulled inward into isolation, trapped within her torpor and forced to face the acidic gnaw of her head pain. Rich, hating any and all silence, was uncomfortable and flustered by not having a distraction. He shuffled his sandaled feet and dug deep into the pockets of his khakis, searching for money that he may have forgotten about that could have gone through the wash; any bit of luck to cling to.

"Hey, remember that one Halloween when you guys dressed up last minute?" asked Rich, having found not a cent in his pockets, but stumbling upon a memory instead.

Steph raised her eyebrows, surprised by her father's pull.

"Yeah, maybe," said Steph. "I remember Mom saying that she wouldn't pay for store-bought costumes, and so we made them."

"I've always thought that store-bought costumes were soulless," said Lisa. "Wouldn't you rather have something that you put a bit of yourself into?"

"We scrounged through our closets," said Rich. "We were trying to piece something together. And that's when Josh came up with the idea to go as-"

"As a guy carrying a head!" Steph yelled so loud that Lisa winced.

"That's right!" said Rich. "Josh wore my flannel jacket and, because you were shorter of course (only coming up to his chest), you climbed inside and stuck your head out of the middle of the buttoned-up jacket. You rested your head in his hands, and it looked, kind of, like he was carrying your head."

"We even did my face up to look like it was decapitated," Steph chuckled. "Bloody mouth, bloody nose, grey in the face. Mom did a really great job."

"I used to do my all of my sisters' makeup for Halloween. We'd go as *The Munsters* every year," said Lisa, rubbing her temple but trying to engage.

"And you guys waddled up the block," said Rich. "You had to walk in unison. It was hilarious. I said, 'Why don't you guys just separate and then reform in front of the next house?' But Josh was adamant that you guys walk together, stay in character. Finally, you gave up. It was too difficult to walk in unison, but also people weren't really getting it; you kept having to explain the costume. When you told him that you wanted to walk alone, Josh was absolutely pissed. 'What do we go as if we're not together?' And you said-"

"'I'll go as a dead person because I look dead.' And he said, 'What about me?' And I said, 'You can be a poor person because Dad's flannel doesn't fit and it makes you look poor.'"

They laughed, Rich buckling over to slap his knee.

"It made no sense," said Steph. "And it was very cruel, but it felt right in the moment."

"He was absolutely pissed," said Rich. "For the rest of the night, he pouted from house to house. But I think he was less upset with you and more upset at the lack of creativity."

"Do you remember when he decided to stop trick-or-treating?" asked Steph. "You guys dressed up and handed out candy."

"We dressed up as clowns. I let him do my makeup. It wasn't half bad. He was my 'assistant.' Kids would knock on the door, and I'd say, 'Hey there, boys and girls. Would you like some candy? Let me call over my assistant, Bee-Bo.' And I'd honk my nose, and he'd come waddling in. Again, it was fun for the first few kids, but he just insisted that we keep it up for the whole night. He had a way of hooking to an idea and never letting it go."

"What struck me as so odd," said Lisa, startling Rich and Steph with her inclusion. "Is that Rich was in such good shape. You were very muscular, hun, because you had been training cadets at the time, so the kids would ring the bell and when the door opened there was this clown who looked like he was on steroids. Frankly, I was surprised they didn't find it terrifying."

"The vast majority of the children were frightened and confused, yes," said Rich.

The family sat in the silence of remembrance, a melange of memory revolving through their heads, mixing together as if each individual memory had grown to such a size, like an expanding atom, they began to conflate and soak into the physical world. They felt too big to contain and held such great power that it felt as if they could persuade their fragile reality that they were not where they were.

"But he could get grumpy," said Steph, uncomfortable with the power they were giving her brother.

"He could," said Rich with tacit understanding.

"He had a bit of a temper if he didn't get his way," said Lisa, also getting it.

"We had to take his video games away because he got way too into them," said Rich. "He was playing this duck hunting game on his Nintendo, and he was so into it that he would scream, 'Die! Die! Die!' at some of the birds. I was like, 'Okay, I think we've had enough of this, buddy.' I took it away and hid it up in the closet. He screamed, 'I hate you!' and didn't come out of his room for dinner."

"Remember when you bought him that jacket?" asked Lisa with a mischievous smirk.

"I stand by that jacket," said Rich, the scab of a raw wound having been ripped off.

"He looked ridiculous in it," said Lisa, laughing. "We were new in Evanston, and you took him to Kohl's for back-to-school shopping and bought him a leather jacket. 'Wear this on the first day. Everyone will think you're the coolest guy in school,' you told him. He looked like a Fonzarelli impersonator. Just awful."

Steph watched Rich and Lisa share their laugh.

"He came home from school," said Rich. "And I was like,

'How'd it go, bud?' And he said, 'First period someone said, 'Hey Goose, where's Maverick?!' He threw the jacket in the garbage and was pissy with me for a month."

"He was such a brat when we moved to Evanston," said Lisa.

"You're telling me," said Steph. "We had only been there a month, and I was having trouble making friends. I went up to him during lunch, hoping to sit with him, and he acted like he didn't know me. He accused me of 'cramping his style.'"

"That's awful!" said Lisa. "That doesn't sound like him at all."

"He just wanted to fit in. I get it," said Steph, wanting to extenuate the blow she had landed on her helpless brother.

"When I told him we were moving from Oregon to Evanston, he was furious," said Lisa. "He was going to miss all of his friends, he said. We had already moved around so much with Rich's career, and the last thing we wanted to do was pull you kids out of there. You were both so comfortable. He was so upset, crying every day after school. When I tried to talk to him about it he exploded at me, 'You have no idea what it's like! You didn't move around when you were a kid! You have no idea what it's like!' And he had his finger in my face, and I just snapped. I slapped his finger away, and I slapped him."

"Lisa. You didn't mean to."

"It was the slightest tap. I was so angry. I swear, it was so light, it was mostly to startle him. And it did. He bawled and apologized. I did as well. But still, I..." Throbbing. As if her head was in a vice. She winced, her pinched brow bringing her gaze to the floor.

Rich sensed that maybe this was a sign that they had reminisced enough. The memories had dissipated with Lisa's crumbling state, perhaps symbolizing that it was best to plant themselves firmly in the present.

"I'm going to get some fresh air," said Rich, clapping his hands together as if he were a college football coach having just finished an inspirational speech. A job well done. Before he could leave the room, Lisa reached for him.

"I think I'm dehydrated," said Lisa. "Give me some of your emergency water."

He smiled, handing it to her, then walked out of the room.

Rich walked the halls of the hospital. He noticed the patients in various stages of their treatments. A woman in a wheelchair, probably in her late eighties, was being pushed by a nurse.

"I want a blanket," she said.

"You have a blanket, Eileen."

"Oh. Is this the same one you gave me for my birthday?"

"Yes," said the nurse, unsure how to answer.

The inevitability that Rich will be in a situation similar to Eileen bothered him, but he quickly shrugged it off. He had contemplated death all his life, but this was always his tactic when faced with insuperable fate. In the military, he prepared men to live. If they listened to him, completely, if they diligently executed their pushups and their crunches and their pull-ups, meeting the physical standards that the United States Army required, they could be strong enough to escape death. This ideology had penetrated Rich's psyche, inveigling him to believe that if he could wrench himself into the form of a task-driven, myopic soldier, he could defeat the existential enemy. The oblivion was a villain, a rapacious dictator who took what he wanted without asking why. The malevolent ruler possessed an entire kingdom, but it would never get Rich.

He walked out the automatic doors and stood in the autumnal world of decomposing leaves. A brisk breeze brushed off the wet grass. Fall had firmly arrived. He inhaled deeply but breathed the rank stench of cigarette smoke and old potpourri. It was the fragrance of his mother. Someone the dictator had taken long ago. He looked to his left where a woman Rich's age smoked.

"You can bum one if you want," she said. "But they're Camel Lights."

"Oh, that's okay. I don't smoke."

Her smile faded, feeling judged. She nodded and stared deep into the wet pavement of the hospital parking lot. Rich stared with her, happy to be sharing a moment with his mother again. The sliding, automated doors behind him opened as visitors and ex-patients left. He enjoyed watching this. It was similar to being at the airport, watching people come home to family and significant others. He saw a young woman, probably early twenties, limping on crutches. She was assisted by, what Rich assumed was, her fiancé. This most likely being the case as she was wearing a ring and the boy was not. A friend had the car pulled up front. He leaped from the front seat with sprightly energy, both of the young men helping her into the front seat of the car. It meant a lot to the young woman that they were there for her. This was an enormous episode in their young lives. Another couple exited. They reminded Rich of him and Lisa. The wife rubbed the back of the husband's neck as the man winced, his arm in a sling. She whispered something funny to him, which he laughed at but winced again.

Someone else exited. It was someone he recognized, but couldn't quite place at first. A man in his thirties, leaving with a young boy. It was the father he had spoken to several days ago. Gone was the baseball uniform. The father's hand rested on his boy's shoulder, who walked very gingerly, clutching his lower abdomen. The father ruffled the boy's hair, then, upset that there was anything else out of place on his boy, smoothed it back into place. The father looked over his shoulder, feeling Rich's eyes. They smiled at one another, the father throwing a thumbs-up as if to say, "All is well." Rich returned the thumbs-up with enthusiasm. The father and son descended into the parking lot. He watched them with the woman who smelled like his mother until they were out of sight.

CHAPTER FIFTEEN

JOSH AND HIS GANG OF UNHINGED FRIENDS STAGGERED
down the vacant streets of a city blanketed in the rich hues of
sunset. Josh's shoulder was jammed, and his breathing
labored, betokening a fracture somewhere within his torso.
Every breath unleashed ravenous bites to his nervous system
as if his skin were covered in a swarm of psychotic ants. His
face pulsed in unison with his heartbeat as he stuffed cocktail
napkins up his nose in an effort to halt the bleeding. Nausea
rippled throughout his torpid muscles, the beer in his gut
questioning whether or not it belonged. His gait was a dragging of his back foot, like that of a disfigured ogre trudging
forth with little joy or energy.

Making things worse was the indecorous mood of his
intoxicated friends. The group spread themselves throughout
the wide streets, taking up as much space as they could; a
post-apocalyptic street gang. They drank from bottles of
booze they stole from a liquor store and upon completion,
smashed them in the street. Josh felt ill-at-ease as the battered
buildings stared down at them like judgmental statues as his

anarchic friends raged with drunken fury. Just ahead, Bruno and Big Boy Bear walked with one another, emphatically free-style rapping. Bruno drunkenly beat-boxed, his spittle flying through the air as he danced in a circle with the spastic energy of a broken sprinkler. Big Boy Bear drunkenly improvised lazy gangsta rap:

"Yo, I'm so ill /
Mufuckas know I pop bottles like pills /
Push me bitch and you find out that I kills /
Cuz I got hoes in the valleys and tha hills /
Bitch, wachoo want? I'm so fuckin raw /
I goes hawd /
I fuck you up bad, you be screaming out 'Oh, lawd!'"

The lines were a blathering annoyance that refused to let up. Behind Josh, Lonny walked with Natalie, his arm around her, pushing himself on his tip-toes to put his tongue in her ear. She laughed maniacally, amplifying her pleasure when Josh turned around to look. It only encouraged Lonny's aggressive intentions as he groped her for the world to see.

Keira walked beside Josh, but she didn't seem to notice him, or anyone else for that matter. She had a distant look in her cloudy eyes, zombified as she strode next to him mechanically.

"Why didn't you tell him to stop?" Josh asked her with the altered voice of someone with something up their nose.

She didn't answer. She smiled and nodded in recognition, seeing something up ahead. Josh looked to see what she had seen, but there was nothing. Andy handed Josh another cocktail napkin, which he took, replacing and tossing away the strawberry-red bulb he had crammed into his left nostril.

"Man. Dewey really went to town," said Andy.

"Mhm."

"No. I mean, like. He really enjoyed himself. Really took his time."

"Yeah."

"But you held in there. Not in the way that like, you put up a fight or anything. I mean, I was more shocked that you stayed conscious for as long as you did."

"Me too."

"Because, like I said, he really went after you. He got into a rhythm pretty quickly, and he just stayed in it. Just, bam, bam, bam, pause to catch his breath, then bam, bam, bam."

"Okay, Andy."

"Sorry, Joshy. Want another napkin?"

"No." He checked the one he'd just put up his nose. It was soaked. "Never mind. Yes." Andy handed him a napkin along with an empathetic furrowing of his brow.

The streets were mysteriously empty except for wind-blown litter and fleeing herds of rats. Occasionally, someone would run through the streets, their briefcase or purse tucked under their arm, the rats scampering about their feet. The dashing patrons reminded Josh of the midwest streets when Chicago citizens saw an encroaching storm. The clouds would radiate with green, the humidity solidifying, panic amongst the city slowly building. It always felt as if a bomb were about to hit. An ominous tone clung to the air like a sour radio wave; a poorly tuned power chord from a garage sale guitar.

The buildings were vestigial versions of themselves, some having lost windows, others decorated with half-finished spray paint tags. The once Panglossian streets had wizened into the dregs of 1970's New York. The asphalt of the city streets bubbled in disrepair, congruous to the winding River

Styx as it snaked through the rotting shores of dilapidated buildings.

But no matter the morose site, Josh's group took their time, meandering as they drank, celebrating themselves. Every minute was punctuated with a newly smashed bottle and a cry from Lonny, "Fuck yeah!" Natalie cackled and applauded every shatter like fireworks over Lake Michigan. Josh was exhausted and wished for an alternative route to somewhere, anywhere, just as long as it was far away from these people and this place.

"Josh?... Josh Husk?"

A weak voice lofted the question from the gutter. A gaunt man, disheveled and sinewy, sat on the curb, wrapped in stitched-together rags. He looked like a beleaguered old friar who was in the midst of a defiant hunger strike. As he slowly rose to his feet, Josh recognized the man.

"Mr. Flynn?"

"You remember," said Mr. Flynn, his face flooding with joy.

"Of course! Third grade! You were one of my most favorite teachers."

They embraced. Josh felt the bones under the thick rags, Mr. Flynn's weak arms barely being able to grasp tightly to Josh. He smelled of mold and urine.

"Wow, that's wonderful to hear, Josh. It warms my heart, you have no idea how tremendous it is to hear that."

"Do you remember the science fair? I did a presentation on citric electricity, and how many grapefruits you would need to power a living room. Do you remember that? I put my heart and soul into that thing."

"Ha! Yes. Of course, I do. You were always such a wonderful student. One of my very best. So creative."

The gang of stumbling miscreants had moved beyond

them, the sounds of shattering bottles being heard in the distance like the howling of coyotes.

"You were always such a kind boy," said Mr. Flynn. "You brought the best out of all of the other students. Never without a friend."

"Yeah, I guess I did have a lot of friends back then. It was easier to like people, I suppose."

"No, no, no. You were always so wonderful."

"Well, thanks, Mr. Flynn."

"Is everything all right? You look like you got a little roughed up by someone."

"Oh, yeah. Just a little squabble with an old bully. Um, sorry for saying so, Mr. Flynn, but you don't look so healthy yourself. Everything okay?"

"No, Josh. I'm afraid it isn't. After you left, I fell on some hard times. My health isn't so good."

"That's terrible, sir."

"Yes, well, it's the way it goes sometimes. But seeing you has made me feel so much better. It's miraculous what seeing an old student can do for a teacher. It breathes life into you." Mr. Flynn held out his hand, which Josh took. He felt fragile, his spavined hand feeling as if under the skin were a web of unconnected wires.

"But since I have you, Josh. Would you mind if I asked you for a loan? Just a little something to get me-"

"Hey, you fucking pervert!" yelled Lonny, the gang suddenly swarming upon Mr. Flynn. "Get the fuck away from Josh!"

"No, you guys. This is my old teacher," said Josh, trying to stop the advancing battalion.

"We know who he is," said Lonny. "This dude is a total scumbag."

"Get the fuck away from me, Lonny!" hissed Mr. Flynn, his face turning pointed and reptilian. "I'll fucking kill you!"

Mr. Flynn turned, coiled, weakly brandishing a large buck knife that looked like it had been sharpened on the curb. It was jagged and scratched, sinister looking, but too big for the old man. Lonny quickly kicked the knife out of his hands. It fell to the ground with a pathetic clang.

"You still owe me money, mother fucker," said Lonny, advancing on the man.

"What's going on here?" begged Josh.

"Good ol' Mr. Flynn here is a fucking crack head. He goes around begging people for loans, says he's going to use it for food and what not, but he just ends up spending it on crack cocaine."

"Please, Lonny," said Mr. Flynn. "I swear, just give me a little bit. I swear I'll spend it on food this time."

"You won't get one red fucking cent from me, dude."

Lonny had Mr. Flynn by the throat, pressed against the brick wall of the building behind him and sliding down onto the ground.

"I'll do anything, Lonny," said Mr. Flynn. "I'll... I'll do it, Lonny. I'll suck your dick, Lonny. Please, I'll do it. Just give me a little something. I'll do it."

Josh turned away, repulsed and bewildered. He couldn't watch such a prodigious figure in his mind be reduced to a crack whore. Lonny shoved the old man further into the cement. Big Boy Bear tapped Lonny on his shoulder with a heavy, stuffed paw.

"I've got this, Lonny."

Lonny nodded, backing away to allow Big Boy to take his place.

"No. Please, Big Boy. Have a heart."

A button eye hung from Big Boy's face as his sinister,

stitched grin stretched from ear to ear. He lifted his hulking foot and slammed it into Mr. Flynn. Big Boy stomped down repeatedly as if he were putting out a bag of lit dog shit. The destructive force of the plush, oversized limb didn't seem to do so much damage as one would think, but it was powerful enough to bounce the old man into the hard, cold ground. It pushed him into the pavement, extinguishing life.

Bruno and Natalie pulled the homicidal Big Boy from the defeated pile of rags. Mr. Flynn lay on the ground, a cowering mess, bruised and bloodied. As Andy tugged at Josh's arm to continue on, Josh looked back and thought he saw the old man crack an eye, which relieved him to know that Mr. Flynn was probably playing dead at the feet of the querulous bear.

The newly-formed gang commenced walking the streets as if nothing had happened, in search of other terrors. Bruno had just finished rolling a blunt with a grape swisher he had swiped from the liquor store. Keira perked up, eyeing him as he finished licking the seal.

"That looks good," she said, seductively.

"Yuu wansum?" slurred Bruno.

"Yes, please."

"Have you evr shotgunnd before?"

"No, what is it?"

"Iss like, when you smoke and yuu pass it mouths ta mouth."

"Sounds fun."

Bruno swayed like a tower of poorly stacked bricks as he drunkenly lit the blunt. He inhaled deeply, his eye bulging from their sockets.

"Okay, open yer mouth, close yer eyes," he squeaked through his smoke-filled lungs.

Keira did as he advised. Bruno blew a stream of grey

skunk weed into Keira's awaiting mouth, which was received with blissful grace. As her eyes opened, they erupted in red, her facial muscles slackening. She smiled like a fool.

"Your turn," said Keira.

She took the joint from Bruno and inhaled deeply, much deeper than Bruno. She held the smoke for five seconds like a veteran doper and waved Bruno close. He closed his eyes and opened his mouth. Keira grabbed his shoulders and brought her lips to his, releasing what fumes her lungs possessed into his sucking mouth. His eyes burst open and, with Keira still clinging to his face, stared at Josh in alarm. Josh stood, diffident and unsure of himself. He walked away, trying to imagine he was somewhere else. Andy took notice of his taciturn demeanor.

"What's up, doc?" asked Andy.

"Nothing, man," said Josh. He stopped, noticing they were at the feet of one of the most historic buildings of all time. "Wow, would you look at that? The Empire State Building."

"It's so big," said Natalie.

Lonny whispered something into Natalie's ear. She burst out laughing.

"Oh my god, stop! You're so bad."

"Big Boy. You got that thing I asked you to bring?" asked Andy, suddenly eager.

Big Boy nodded with a stitched, mischievous smile. He reached around to his backside, but struggled.

"Fuckin hell, man. Josh, would you mind helping me out?"

"With what?"

"Unzip me."

Crawling down the middle of Big Boy's back was a zipper hidden amongst the fur. Josh was reluctant, but Big

Boy eyed him expectantly. And seeing how the truculent bear had just stomped his third-grade teacher into submission, Josh reached for the zipper. Slowly, but surely, Josh pulled it southwards. It made an aberrant sound of twisting hide and stretching skin as it ripped the bear's back in two. He reached the zipper's end at the middle of Big Boy's buttocks.

"Okay. You're unzipped."

"Reach inside," grunted the bear.

"Dude, come on."

"Reach inside, Josh. We ain't got all day."

Josh looked to Andy for help, but all he offered was an implicit nod to vouchsafe that he reach inside the stuffed bear. Josh cringed, awaiting the surprise from his friends to notify him that this was all a cruel joke.

Josh eased his hand into the backside of the bear. White stuffing welcomed him and pulled him closer. It undulated, alive and wanting. It gripped his forearm, squeezing it like a woman's orifice when visited by a welcomed intruder. It held to him, squirming with delight as it tugged, jostling his arm.

"Jesus. Take your sweet fucking time, Josh," said the angry bear, lighting a cigarette and puffing with impatience.

As if it were thrust into his hand, Josh felt the object in question: a can. He took it as his invitation for escape. He quickly pulled his hand from the wriggling fluff.

"Bout fucking time."

Josh was confused to see that it was a can of red spray paint.

"Ah! There we are," said Andy, snatching it from Josh's trembling hand.

Josh felt violated by the immensity of the disturbing act, and the fact that the bounty was a meaningless household item made it feel all the more unnerving. Natalie and Lonny stood nearby as Andy popped off the lid and shook the can with rhythm and thoughtful intent.

"Hmm. So many options," said Andy. "Oh! I know."

He unleashed a blood-red stream from the can, diligently tracing the word of choice along the side of the old, respected building. Natalie and Lonny being the closest audience laughed at their sneak preview of Andy's graffiti opus. Andy finally backed away, and Josh could see now that the word was "FUCK."

Natalie and Lonny chuckled like tickled school children. Natalie, suddenly inspired, grabbed the can from Andy and took the building to task. Riding the wave of Andy's creativity, she grasped at the first idea that came to mind and saw to its impetuous completion. "CUNT," it read. This drew laughs and high fives. Big Boy puffed on his cigarette and chuckled, the smoke billowing from his button snout and unzipped spine.

"I got one, I got one," said Lonny as he staggered towards the building. It was apparent that his fast drinking had caught up with him as he was visibly belligerent. He started to scrawl something but stopped as he forgot his word.

"Wait. Fuck, it was... Oh yeah, I remember."

He began again but kept stopping. The fumes from the can were overwhelming and were failing to blend with the booze in his stomach. He paused, taking deep breaths, but this only brought more toxins into his lungs. He belched, his limbs quivering. He gathered himself and pushed through. His word was "BITCASTITS." He stumbled back onto his heels, rocked by the poison vapor.

"What the fuck is that supposed to say?" asked Natalie.

"I don't know, man. I kinda lost my shit while I was doing it."

The gang boomed with laughter as Lonny fell to a knee,

trying to compose himself. The laughter crescendoed with calamitous energy. As the moment swelled, and they locked eyes in a tacit understanding that a physical event was needed to cap off this great success of delinquency.

A crash. Broken glass. Natalie had grabbed a rock from the gutter and thrown it into one of the lower windows. The idea spored, infecting everyone with a want for destruction. They clambered for loose bricks, rocks, and empty beer bottles and hurled them at the building. They shattered windows, broke fixtures, and chipped away at the illustrious exterior of the once esteemed building.

Absent were Bruno and Keira, who Josh found still behind the group, shotgunning smoke into each other's awaiting maws. Josh approached, enraged by the anarchy. He didn't know what he was going to do, but he needed to stop someone from getting what they wanted. Bruno saw Josh and backed away from Keira.

"Loog, man. We were juss smokin. It wuzz nuthin."

Josh tempered his boiling anger.

"It's okay, Bruno."

Bruno nodded, thankfully. He eyed the chaos as if it were a house full of Christmas lights and ran towards it, grabbing a chunk of loose asphalt along the way.

"Come on, Josh," said the dazed, bubbly Keira. "We were just playing around. You know I'm your girl. I'm your girl, Josh."

"Sure. Okay."

"Kiss me, baby."

"Not right now."

"Do it. Kiss me. Kiss me in front of everyone, Josh."

"No. I don't want to."

"Let's go into the alley, Josh. Take me into the alley and fuck me, Josh."

Josh was troubled by her aggressive, lecherous tone. Her eyes were demonic, and it was clear to him that Keira was possessed. Thankfully, a distraction sliced through the satanic tension, which happened to be Lonny vomiting into the gutter. The fumes were too strong for his yawing gut. The sounds of the miscellaneous detritus being launched at the building ceased. The group gathered around Lonny like hyaenas around a wounded gazelle.

"Look at this fucking idiot!" boomed Big Boy Bear.

"I thought you were supposed to be a fucking man?!" laughed Natalie.

"Bro, you don looog too goooood," said Bruno

"Had something bad for lunch, Lonny?" prodded Andy.

Lonny tried to speak, but he couldn't stop vomiting. The horrid site was made worse by the amount that had come crawling upward and at such a feverish pace. Much like the off-putting gaze from Keira, Lonny's retching was the scene from an exorcism. It was an unholy purge that looked to Josh to be the sign of a rising shadow of inescapable menace.

Josh turned, feeling a presence. He spotted a patch of woods. The woods sat across a stretch of meadow where the city stopped abruptly. This grouping of forest was familiar to him as they looked to be the very same woods that rested near his family home in Oregon. He used to ride his bike through the trails, hike with his friends and family. Wonderful memories and welcomed comfort beckoned him forth.

He crossed the street, a dedicated stride leading him to the open field.

"Joshy!" cried Andy. "Where you going, pal?"

"Yeah, we're heading to Bruno's. Josh! His mom's old place, we're gonna throw a kegger," yelled Big Boy.

Josh waved them off. "I don't know why, but I need some fresh air. I'll catch up with you guys later."

The woods were a mixture of elms, oaks, and furs. A conflation of deciduous and evergreen that formed a multilayered, imperturbable universe of serenity. He had to cross the prairie to get there, as it always was, but this was a buffer zone that he greatly enjoyed. In the fall, as it was now, the grass was surging back to life, having been torched from the parched summer. The dead grass formed a pale yellow, while the reinvigorated blades took on a verdant radiancy, causing them to bleed into one another and form a rolling ocean surface that replicated the reflection of a setting sun. Josh sliced through the long blades, the wild strands reaching his waist just as he remembered. A stiff breeze kicked up, pushing him toward the tree line. Above the forest hung a deep swell of portentous clouds. They circled and swirled like angry billows of factory smoke. A slight drizzle prefaced an inevitable storm, its light fuzz laying a thin sheet of rain on his face. As Josh marched forward, through the ocean of rolling grass, Lonny's bodily functions faded into the distance. The trees grew closer.

CHAPTER SIXTEEN

THEY WAITED FOR THE DOCTOR. STEPH SAT IN HER SAME chair, her back to the window, facing into the middle of the room. Rich maintained his leaned position against the wall, his tan arms crossed in front of his chest, foot tapping nervously at a rhythmic, frenetic pace to indicate his inner turmoil. Lisa was seated next to the bed, rubbing her aching brow in the hopes of massaging the right blood vessel that would open the floodgates, allowing a rush of blood to her brain that would assuage her searing migraine. Josh was where he had been for some time.

They had all received a call from a nurse that Dr. Kaspin would like to speak with them. The request was poorly timed as Steph had finally managed to pull herself away, albeit for emergency sustenance; i.e., she went to McDonald's for lunch. She hadn't had a meal from the establishment since she was a child. Actually, that's not true. The last time she had anything from McDonald's was in the Phoenix airport when she and Shawn were returning from their honeymoon in Costa Rica, and they had a layover in Arizona at one in the morning, and McDonald's was the only restaurant that was open. Either way, the choice to eat at McDonald's was always a decision born from desperation. She caved, craving the gluten and fat she had been avoiding for so long. Fortuitously, there was one positioned across the street from the hospital; she could see it from her window. Steph had ventured over and was enraged when she ordered a Big Mac (no cheese), but was handed a Happy Meal by mistake.

"I'm sorry, but I didn't order this."

"Oh. Well, that's what it says on the receipt."

"Why would I, a grown adult, order a Happy Meal?"

"I don't know. Maybe you have a kid?"

The attendant started to walk away, but Steph brought her back.

"Okay, but then why wouldn't I have ordered food for myself? Why would I only order one meal for a child?"

"What?"

"I'm saying why would I just order a meal for a kid? The flaws in your excuse are very apparent."

"Look, do you want me to swap it out? I mean, it's basically the same thing."

"What do you mean? How can it be the same thing? You handed me a kid's meal."

"It's the same thing, Mam. There's a double cheeseburger in there, no cheese, it has the same amount of calories as the burger in the adult meal. You ordered a small fry, and there's a medium in there. You get a package of cookies on top of it. Not to mention a free toy. If you're asking me, I'd just take it and walk away."

Steph sat in her respective chair, next to the opened window with the fall breeze blowing in. She flicked a fidget spinner, which had come as the toy in the Happy Meal. It whirred as it spun in circles, spinning and spinning, a propeller propelling nothing, going nowhere. She marveled at its lack of purpose, and yet it fulfilled its empty existence so perfectly. She felt at ease as she flicked it. It spun and spun, making a ratcheting whir that caused Rich to stare, hypnotized as well. Lisa rubbed her temples, annoyed.

"Please, Stephanie. Please. Stop it."

Dr. Kaspin entered with the gait of a professional who was all business; he radiated dire sincerity. Steph pocketed her toy, Rich's bouncing foot ceased, and Lisa's migraine was silenced as they became an attentive audience, attempting to interpret every move Dr. Kaspin made, agog to obtain any inkling of tone that his posture would possess.

"Afternoon, everyone. Thank you for getting here so quickly. I would like to give you as much information as I can, and I will, but it can get a little complicated. I know there will be questions, so please tell me if I'm going too fast."

They nodded. Someone, Steph wasn't sure, either Rich or Lisa mumbled, "So, how is he?"

"Not well. I'm afraid that, as we had spoken about earlier, there was damage to the rear of the brain, the parietal lobe and the occipital lobe. The damage was compounded by the bleeding from the burst blood vessel, and although we did everything we could with surgery, he hasn't been responding to the reflex tests. Which is, to be frank, not good at all. I'm afraid that during his accident there was a type of damage done that is called 'axonal shearing,' which is a series of tears in the tissues of the brain between the cells."

"How did you not spot these before?" asked Steph. "Why is this the first time we're hearing about this?"

Dr. Kaspin was surprised, not by the question, just by its source. He had been watching in Lisa's direction, awaiting stiff rebuke or a firm line of questioning. But he noticed that his suspected adversary was quietly listening, seated in the corner with a sallow face, staring at the linoleum floor. Steph had taken charge.

"Well, it's the kind of damage that reveals itself over time," said Dr. Kaspin. "It's common in most mild to traumatic head injuries, and it's a process we can't halt. Damage to the axons in the brain can exponentially worsen in the following days, leading to a breakdown in communication between neurons. The axons degenerate, releasing toxic chemicals called neurotransmitters into the extracellular space. In turn, many of the surrounding neurons die off, and this is a process that can increase rapidly within the space of as little as forty-eight hours. This, of course, exacerbated the initial effects of Josh's injury."

Steph searched for a question but instead elected to nod for the Doctor to continue.

"Josh has what we've labeled a Diffuse Axonal Injury, or DAI. Comas are typical, but with his bleeding episode, and the persistence of his vegetative state, we're going to recommend artificial nutrition, along with mechanical ventilation."

"Life support," said Lisa with a weak sigh.

"Yes," said Dr. Kaspin. "Now this is where you may want to have a discussion amongst your family of what might be the best option for Josh, and for yourselves. We cannot encourage the stopping or withdrawing of tube feeding, so this should be a decision that you come to as a group."

"What's the possibility that, if we began the treatment, he could come out of it?" asked Steph.

"Low. Some people do come out, but very, very rarely. In most cases, this is a measure performed to merely extend their life, or the dying process, only until other systems in the body begin to fail. Long term coma patients, ones with Josh's severe wounds, do on the rarest of occasions come out of it. However, they bring with them some side effects and permanent problems. They'll have poor muscle control. They can be very uncooperative, many suffer from severe depression. They may also require extensive in-home care if it's permitted safe for them to even be outside of a facility."

"So he'd never be the same again?" asked Rich, no longer leaning.

"It's highly doubtful. Or-"

"Or..." said Steph.

"Or, if the family agrees to it, we can begin comfort care. We can allow things to take their natural course, making him as comfortable as possible. I assure you, besides these options, we have done our very best. I can also assure you that, if you decide to go with comfort care, it would not be in vain as Josh is an organ donor. So-"

"Okay, sorry, but I think we need-"

"Yes, forgive me. Needless to say, there are some things to consider. And a decision does not need to be made at this very moment. Please, take some time. But we will need to know in the next couple of days, for if you do elect to put him on assisted nutrition and ventilation, we'd like to begin that treatment immediately. I have some pamphlets here, along with some of the paperwork that I'll leave by the door. You can acquaint yourselves with them in your own time. A nurse can also help you with any further details."

They sat in a wake of stillness as Dr. Kaspin realized he was no longer needed or wanted. His job was complete.

"Best of luck to you folks, and my sincerest condolences."

As he left, Steph stared at her mother, searching for signs of life. She sat, scrupulously smoothing the wrinkles in her skirt.

"Tell me what you're thinking, Mom," demanded Steph.

"I don't know, Stephanie."

"What's going through your head right now? At this moment."

"I said, I don't know. And I'd rather not talk for a minute."

"Bullshit. You want to pull the plug."

"My goodness, please, Stephanie," said Lisa with a painful cringe. "I haven't the slightest clue what we should do. The doctor hasn't been out the door for two minutes. Now just stop it-"

"What about you, Dad?" asked Steph.

Rich heaved a sigh, his barrel chest rising and collapsing. "I just want Josh back. I want Josh to be back and to be himself. But from the sounds of things, that doesn't seem like much of an option."

"Oh my god, you're both giving up!" Steph boomed as she shot to her feet. She stood in the middle of the room, commanding the space like a valorous chess piece which had captured the center of the board. Rich and Lisa snapped their eyes toward her, shocked by her fury.

"You're giving up when he needs us most! You heard the doctor: it's rare. But there's still a chance! Isn't that enough?"

"He wouldn't be himself," said Lisa. "I've seen this, Stephanie. If they come out of this, which is a huge if, they're not much different from the how they were when they were in it. They're still vegetative. If Josh came back he would be incapable of taking care of himself. This is a decision that demands serious thought. And right now I'm just not sure."

"Well, now is not the time to be flighty, Mom. To me, the choice is obvious. He's still here. He's still Josh. How can you give up on him if there's still even the slightest sliver of hope?"

She was expecting a fight from the often pugnacious matriarch. It was unlike her to not return with a barbarous blow, defending her position no matter what it was, right or wrong. No matter the conflict, she was always prepared to exchange, and hell-bent on winning. But she merely fidgeted in silence.

"I'll be gone in twenty years," said Lisa, finally.

"Jesus, Mom."

Steph thought her iconoclast use of her mother's savior's name would stir outrage, but instead Lisa kept a controlled tone.

"Say he comes out of it. Then your father and I go. Then what? What happens to Josh?"

"I'll take care of him."

"You have a son. You have a husband; your own life. A career. How could you bear it?"

"I'll do whatever it takes. Shawn and Levi would help out."

"You'd put Levi through that?"

"Don't, Mom."

"You have enough to worry about in your own life. We never see or hear from you. You only call on birthdays and holidays, you won't come and see us for longer than an afternoon, and you can't wait to leave when you do. You're short and judgmental the entire time. Your marriage is in jeopardy. You've neglected your job. So please tell me: how can you take care of Josh if you can't take care of yourself?"

There she was as she knew her. Contemptuous and coiled, eager for scornful reproach. But as soon as she had erupted, she withered away in capitulation, her menace giving way to enveloping lassitude.

"I'm sorry," said Lisa. "We won't sign anything unless we've all come to an agreement. I didn't mean those things. I'm just tired, and my head is killing me."

"Right. Well..." Steph had nothing left.

Standing in the middle of the room now felt absurd and needless, but Steph couldn't bring herself to sit. She didn't want to leave the room either. She was sweaty and claustrophobic. Her stance was wide and ready, her fingers wiggling through the air, demanding the fidget spinner. But if she returned to the toy, she'd feel judged as a child, incapable of making a decision of such importance and weight. Instead, she crossed to the window, undoing the lock on the pane.

"What are you doin', kiddo?" asked Rich.

"Opening the window. I need some air."

It felt like opening a tomb, cold air rushing into the room, replacing the stuffy negativity with the breeze of an oncoming storm. A steady blanket of rain splattered onto the pavement outside, cracking thunder booming in the distance. Steph reached her hand out, allowing the water to trickle down her palm and wrist. She stared at the McDonald's across the street, its drive-thru filled with customers who were probably getting everything they wanted.

CHAPTER SEVENTEEN

You are running away. There is little choice, as you see it. Terror has ballooned to such an unfathomable size, and you feel so completely bewildered that you didn't realize you were running until you were already deep into the woods.

This is the right decision, you tell yourself. Your old life is behind you now. Your future is ahead, whatever that may be; you haven't the slightest clue, but you are sure that it begins in these woods. They have always provided you with an escape, and now they are acting as your proverbial exit door.

The storm is here. The rain beats on the canopy above like the rolling of a thousand microscopic snare drums, a percussion section of a celestial marching band reverberating from above. The canopy shields most of the downpour, but also causes the water to pool, formulating heavy raindrops with the proportions of atomic bombs; their thunderous boom is felt when they smack onto your forehead as you run amongst the trees. You're having trouble getting solid footing, stumbling as the soil continuously gives way, breaking apart from its overindulgence of liquid. The soil dissolves beneath your feet like an Alka Seltzer tablet submerged in bedside water.

The elephantine trees of elm, oak, and pine loom over you like the legs of giants born from fairy tales, watching as you dart beneath them. You don't have time to look up. You leap over downed logs, ferns, and slick rocks. All the energy you have is being spent on propelling your tired body forward.

It's because he's after you. The figure. He's stalking you, lumbering as he trudges through the gravel and mud. He is nowhere to be seen, only heard. He is somewhere in these woods. Behind you, you believe. You hear his moan in the distance, cutting through the snaring rain and whipping wind. Yes, he is undoubtedly behind you. No matter your efforts, the figure has somehow managed to keep pace.

You white-knuckle the air as you grasp at nothing, using your clenched fists to force blood away from your core and into your legs. Your chest burns like a smoldering campfire. Water and sweat have congealed, fusing into a firm coat of slime that keeps you slippery and makes you feel amphibian. Your legs are emptied of energy and blood, merely boney dowels that stab into the earth, occasionally buckling at the uneven surface. Exhaustion massages your muscles, inveigling them to weaken and concede. Another moan. Closer. A hand has hold of your panicked heart, squeezing.

You have to see. He can't be as close as he sounds. You stop to confront your expectations. So that maybe your worst fears will be staved off. He isn't there. He is nowhere. You wipe your salt-stained eyes, the focus of your vision fuzzy. You listen for a moan, but there is nothing.

The crunch of gravel and sand. The snapping of dead branches. The shuffle of his trudging steps. He has caught up with you, coming towards you from the side, upon you before you can move. He moans, reaching for you as his purple fingers paw at the air. His jaw is open, and his eyes are white. His throat is dry, the groan hoarse and desperate.

You inhale deeply, your limbs bursting to life after receiving an injection of fiery adrenaline. It has unlocked a gear previously thought unavailable to you. At this panicked pace, tears are now added to your macerated hide. You slip through the trees when you eye a large redwood ahead. You make a snap decision, choosing to use it as a hiding place. Maybe he won't see. Maybe he'll come shuffling past, and you can wait until he's gone.

But as you round the massive trunk, you bump into the cold, weak chest of the man. Saul, your grandfather. He wears his hospital robe, which wafts in the breeze. He stands motionless. His catheter and IV dangle, still attached to his bilious skin. He stares at you for a moment, the fog of his eyes cycloning, impregnable in their stormy vacancy. He grabs your shoulders, clinging to you, unable to speak. He inhales deeply, then moans with a deafening rasp. The muscles on his face expand. You can see the broken capillaries that have stretched across his face like a crimson fishnet. He trembles, but with the strength of another world as he shakes you. His sinewy muscles flex as he brings you close. You're coming with him.

But you struggle free, standing for a moment. You shout his name, backing away, but he only plods towards you. Your back makes contact with a surface, but it isn't tree-like. As you turn, you see another golem. Aunt Dotty, your father's sister. She had succumbed to the same tragic illness. Cigarette smoke billows from her nose like a dragon as she looks down at you. She's wearing her infamous skull cap, the one your dad got her when she lost her hair. She grabs your collar and whispers angry, indecipherable susurrus into your face, the same way she did when you wouldn't settle down at her house, or when you yammered too loudly in her hospital room. You try to push her away, but she is determined.

You utilize your wet coat to squirm away, but another decrepit body stumbles over a fallen tree. Your mother's old friend from nursing school, Chris. That thing happened to him with his car. It had been such a random accident. Mom said he was "t-boned." You didn't know what that meant, but it conjured up so many strange, frightening images.

Chris crawls towards you, his neck twisted with jagged metal protruding from his skin.

Then they all come. All of the ones you have forgotten. The forest is filled with the nameless beings as they stumble forward with outstretched arms, reaching for you. You stumble backward and fall to the wet earth. The figures inch closer, Saul leaning over you with his raspy, cold breath. The hands of the others slither from the ground below. They grab you and hold tight at your flailing ankles, wrists, arms, and shoulders. You're pinned to the moist soil as the rain finds its way through the canopy. The vestigial faces of the familiar fill your vision as they pile atop your writhing body. They embrace you, smothering. Once upon you, their bodies relax and slacken. Their weight feels like cinderblocks stacked upon your chest. You try to breathe, but they're much too heavy.

Finally, the weight transfers to the whole of your being as the figures dissolve. They taste of ash but quickly darken into soil. One-by-one they pile and embrace, crumbling into the earth's crust. You sink deeper and deeper, slowly watching the grey sky vanish. The rain is gone, and so is the cold. Warmth fills your body as you are held firmly. As you become one with the forest floor, you take note of the smattering of branches that obscure the sky. The grey of the clouds, the verdant green of the branches with their limbs of dark brown, and the speckled black that is oncoming. You feel your last bit of cold as you fall with the others, entangled in a mesh of past and future.

CHAPTER EIGHTEEN

Steph covered Josh with a thick, wool blanket. It was a typical "Army" blanket: dark green, dense wool, devoid of patterns, and incredibly warm. It had been a gift to Steph from Josh one Christmas; an inside joke, as most of their gifts were. The reference stemmed from their father's obsession with John Wayne. He owned every movie on VHS, along with several made-for-TV documentaries that he had recorded on VCR. Sadly, their video collection consisted of not much else other than the wry cowboy and his broad stage punches. Thusly, they were forced to spend their rainy weekends pilfering their father's sparse film collection, and watching The Duke reign victorious time and time again. But they always marveled at the gear Wayne and his rag-tag crew would pack on horseback. They had canteens, mugs, plate wear, guns, ammunition, and even blankets, all of this equipment wrapped up tightly in their saddlebags. Steph would remark that although the men were always rugged and tough, they also seemed to enjoy snuggling up to a warm campfire.

"They look so cozy!" she'd say.

Josh decided that they could make their own "cowboy beds." They took all the blankets in the house and made camp on the floor in front of the television, and watched The Duke and his cozy friends drift off to dreamland. When Steph had unwrapped the heavy, green Army blanket that Christmas, she knew exactly what it was.

"You got me a cowboy blanket!"

"That's right there, partner," Josh had said in his best Wayne impersonation.

What once was a gift from Josh, was now a gift for Josh. Steph heard the pitter-patter of rushed, short steps as they ran behind her. She knew who it was immediately. She didn't even have to wait for the ensuing hug around her legs.

"Mom, it's raining so hard!"

Levi was drenched, sopping wet.

"Honey, you're soaked."

"Dad had trouble finding parking."

As if on cue, Shawn sauntered into the room, somehow wetter than Levi, wearing a Duke grin of his own. Rich followed behind him, sipping from a newly purchased soda.

"The garage was full, can you believe it?" said Shawn. "We had to walk a block and a half."

"I told him that he should've parked at the Jewel Osco," said Rich. "Rock star parking over there. We got a deal with the assistant manager. Helluva guy. Name is Drew. His father was in the Marines. We had loads to talk about."

Steph lifted Levi into her arms, feeling his soaked clothes press into her dry ones. She hugged him tightly, squeezing him so hard that she felt him squirm to be put back down.

"I'm so glad you're here, munchkin," said Steph.

"Me too, Mom. Is that..." the boy stopped, confused as to whether the body in the bed was his uncle or a nameless corpse.

"Yeah. That's Uncle Josh."

Levi stood firmly, holding a small toy truck. His feet were adorably pigeon-toed as he stared at his unconscious uncle. Steph thought, immediately, they had made a mistake bringing him here.

"Grandpa, have you seen my truck?" said Levi, snapping out of it and showing Rich his small off-road toy that he clutched to, proudly. Steph relaxed, acknowledging she misjudged the moment.

"Wow, now that is cool," said Rich. "How'd you get your hands on something so awesome? Your dad get that for ya?"

"Yeah, he got it for me if he made me promise... oh."

"Made you promise what?" asked Steph.

"I saw Dad smoke," he said. "But don't worry, he's stopping for real this time."

"Yeah, for real this time," said Shawn, trying to play his relapse off jovially.

"Do I still get to keep the truck, Dad?"

"Sure thing, bud. You tried."

"Mom. Everyone from class made a card for Uncle Josh." Levi dropped his backpack to the floor, unzipping it and rifling through. He pulled out a card decorated heavily in marker, illegible to the adult, human eye. It looked like a vomited rainbow. "Kids at school want to know if he's going to be okay. Is he?"

"We'll have to see, hun."

"Dad said he would be."

Steph glowered at Shawn, what the fuck? Shawn shrugged, my bad.

"Hey, I got an idea," said Rich. "Let's see how that truck of yours handles in the rec room. I saw a couple of ramps that would be tailor-made for it."

"Okay, Grandpa. But it can also fly, so you should know that too."

"Got it," he said, nodding to Shawn and Steph, you kids take all the time you need. This obvious gesture annoyed Steph as her father had gotten worse in his old age when it came to hiding his transparency. They shuffled out of the room, Levi launching the truck through the air, fluttering his lips to signify invisible propellers.

"You told him he'd get better? Why the hell would you do that?" asked Steph.

"I didn't know what to tell him. I was shaving, and he kept asking me, and I got a phone call from work, and it just slipped out. He clung to it, man."

"You have to be careful, Shawn. That's what they do. Cling to stuff. And you're smoking again?"

"I know, but that was a couple days ago. I'm back on the patch. It was one, momentary lapse, I swear. I didn't even buy a pack, it was a bummed cig. I can show you the credit statement. I swear, Steph."

She moved back to her chair, which was a chair she was actually beginning to like. She'd been there so long that she thought her spine was conforming to the curve.

"So hey," said Shawn, suddenly excited. "Remember how every year my brother would get us Cheesecake Factory gift cards for Christmas and we'd immediately lose them? Well, I found them! And it turns out they amounted to $185! I took the boy, and we feasted."

"Wonderful."

"And I got you the filet and two slices of cheesecake," he said, digging into a wet to-go bag and proudly presenting his damp offering.

"Two?"

"Yeah, and I know what you're going to say: I can't have

dairy. Well, I remembered this time, and they just so happened to have dairy-free cheesecake! Can you believe it? They had blueberry and strawberry. I got so excited I just got both of them."

Steph dropped her head in her hands. Shawn was taken aback. He did not know her to ever be so outwardly emotional.

"I'm... I'm sorry. I should've known that you liked strawberry better. It's just... well, I tried the blueberry, and it's really good. Well, to be honest. It isn't that good. None of it is that good. I mean, it's fine for a non-dairy product. But I didn't want to go and not get you anything. I at least wanted you to try it."

"No, no. That's fine. It's Josh. They want to-"

"I know. Your dad debriefed me."

"Oh," she said, sniveling and wiping her nose with the sleeve of her college sweatshirt. She felt like hell and looked like she had walking pneumonia. She was dressed in homely, leisure material, head-to-toe. She breathed deeply, finding respite in not having to regale her husband with the current medical drama.

"I brought the old man some apple pie," said Shawn. "He woofed it down before we got to the room."

"He loves Cheesecake Factory," she said, pathetically.

"The size of the menus. It's like, what do you guys do here? Everything? Because maybe you should focus it up a little bit."

"What if we took Josh?"

Shawn was startled but quickly suppressed his reaction. He lifted his eyebrows, but slowly brought them back down. He had been suspecting that this would be a possibility.

"Okay," he said carefully. "So you mean, if he were to

come out of this, you're considering us moving him into the house?"

"Maybe. We could put him in the office. We never really use it."

"That's true. We don't."

Steph was motivated by his reserved demeanor. There was an opening. For this modicum of a moment, she didn't feel insane. This could work, and she had devised a detailed plan for how.

"I could keep working from home. Or, I mean, do a similar thing to what I'm doing now. I talked to Kara, my new supervisor, and she said that they're thinking of opening a new position that would allow me to work from home for most of the week. I'd only need to come into the office on Mondays and Thursdays!"

"That's great." Shawn opened the blueberry cheesecake and searched the wet, brown bag for a fork. His brow was pinched, and his eyes squinted to emulate ponderous thought, indicating that he was seriously considering Steph's idea.

"So I can be home five days out of the week to look after him (which is including weekends)," said Steph. "And his insurance will cover all of his treatment. In some cases, they could pay for a nurse to visit and help on days when I wouldn't be able to be there. Also, there's a government program for people like Josh in which they pay down some of the additional costs for families left with the burden of in-home care. So we'll receive a monthly check, which would be great. And when it comes to food, I've already looked into it, and there's a service that can deliver his meals to our front door every week. We won't ever need to shop for him. And that's just until he can chew. Then it gets a lot easier."

"Sure," said Shawn, taking a bite of cheesecake. He was

hoping the chewing would mean that he wouldn't be expected to answer immediately.

Steph relaxed, catching her breath. She was sweating from the expectation of interruption or an ensuing fight. Shawn always fought her on topics of immediate change or even significant, day-altering plans. Any time Steph had an idea for something as simple as switching out an area of the home decor, Shawn would suddenly grow an affinity for the way she had it. If Steph wanted to leave for a week in January to "escape to someplace warm," Shawn would say that he didn't want to put added pressure on his mom to watch Levi. Steph was sure that her husband wouldn't go for this plan, especially considering the current state of their marriage.

But this had felt different. He was calm and had allowed her to make all of her necessary points. Had she said too much? Now that she had been given the opportunity to say the plan out loud, albeit rushed and cobbled together, she was tentative. It didn't sound like an ideal plan. Perhaps it didn't come out right, or maybe she hadn't articulated it to the best of her ability.

"Speaking of which, how do you like working from home?" said Shawn, thankfully changing the subject. "I mean, working from here. How do you like working from here?"

"It's been okay. To be honest, I haven't gotten much done. My mom seems to be fine one day, then a disaster another. My dad is always in conversation with the open air, waiting for me to chime in."

"I gotta say, that sounds pretty normal."

"Right. And when it comes to Josh, there's been so much changing information, I just want to make sure that I'm here. I've been taking sick days here and there. I've had them stockpiled."

"How many do you have left?"

"Two weeks."

"Oh, cool. So now you just have to avoid getting sick for the rest of the year."

She shot him a look, but she could see that it was in jest. He laughed through a mouthful of cheesecake, his teeth blue from the berries. She softened.

"Yeah. We'll have to start bathing Levi in Purell," she said.

"Oh, we have a whole new bathing routine. Did I not tell you? We ran out of soap, so I've just been putting him in the dishwasher with the pots and pans. The soccer field has been pretty muddy as of late, so I run him on 'heavily soiled.' He comes out shining like a wine glass."

"Oh, soccer! I haven't asked him how he liked his new coach."

"Mrs. Dean, yeah. She's good. She played in college, and the kids just love her. She moved him out of goalie last game, which was a good call because he was just way too scared. If a kid hit a breakaway, I could see him start to crumble. A couple times he just fell to the ground, turtle-shelled. She has him playing defender now, which he loves because all he does is kick the shit out of the ball. Absolutely zero strategy. Just runs up to the fucking thing and wails on it. The kid has a pretty strong leg, Steph. It cracks me up because right after he boots it, he looks to me on the sideline. Like I'm supposed to have something for him. He just booted the thing down-field to the opposing team. He clearly doesn't understand the rules of soccer, which I almost love more than if he were great at it. I don't know what to do, so I just give him a thumbs up. But yeah, kid's got a helluva leg."

Steph stopped a laugh short, submerged in the mist of forgetting something that is too late to mend or recapture.

"Oh my god," she said. "Halloween. I completely missed Halloween!"

"Oh. Uh, yeah."

"You should have told me!"

"I'm pretty sure I did, Steph. I texted you when we were planning on going out, and you said, 'Sounds good.' It's okay, though. It all worked out."

"Oh god, I'm sorry. I wasn't in my right mind. That was-"

"A couple days ago. It was the day you met with Dr. Kaspin. The kid didn't take it personal; he knew vaguely that something important was happening. Or at least, it seemed like he did. But he wasn't upset, we had a great time. Same with everyone at your work, by the way, they're very understanding. I was only messing about the sick days. They'll cut you slack. They all said to tell you hi and give you their best."

"How do you know that?"

"I swooped by to pick up your checks."

"Oh."

She felt as if she had been on another planet. An astronaut who had been selected for a voyage of great distance and importance, but when she came home, she found that the world had rapidly changed. A soldier in war who was getting pieces of information, segments of details on the persistent evolution of life back home. Their lives hadn't frozen, but they had marched on without them. And although they were on the same planet, they felt worlds apart.

"Tell me about Halloween. Please," begged Steph.

"Well, just know that I handled it. I figured your mom wouldn't remind you because, well, you had a ton of shit going on here, but also Jesus isn't involved, so it wasn't going to be on her docket. So, I was very much alone, but I totally nailed it."

"What did he go as?"

"A sea monster."

"What?"

"Yeah, you're telling me. He had been so worried about his uncle, and you of course. I wanted to take his mind off of everything, and I was like, 'What do you want to go as? You can be anything you want, little buddy!' And I'm figuring that means 'store-bought costume,' you know? Like, that's what I would choose if I were a kid. But no, not this kid. He says, 'A sea monster, Dad.'"

"He's been watching that cartoon. The one with the kid who has a friend who's a sea monster. I should've seen that one coming."

"Well, I didn't know that shit. So I'm wracking my brain. I can't tell him no, I just gave him the keys to the kingdom. Far be it from me to take them away just because he's thinking outside the box. So I decide to roll with it. I was like, 'Okay, (you little bastard). You're going as a (fucking) sea monster.' I searched online and didn't find anything, so then I knew that I had to make it. So we went to the craft store-"

"Oh my god. I'm picturing you and him in a craft store, and I'm loving every second of it. Continue."

"I'll have you know: I acclimated quickly. I was perusing fabrics."

"Perusing! Love it."

"I was perusing glitter options. Perusing buttons. A lady came over to help me out."

"I bet she did."

"Oh yeah. Gladys was a real knockout."

"Gladys could easily be a modern hipster name. She was twenty-one, wasn't she?"

"During the Bay of Pigs, yes. So, I told spicy Gladys that I was trying to make my son into a sea monster, and that opened a whole pandora's box of ideas inside of Gladys's

Cold War-era mind. I mean, this hot bitch would not shut up about the time she made this costume for so-and-so grand-daughter, and the time she made that one costume for this grandson-or-other. She has all of these ideas, and we settle on a basket full of materials. And I'll admit. I got inspired."

"Gladys did it for you."

"Oh yeah. Big time. Gladys gave me a full-on creativity erection. She got the motor going. I went home and put this costume together in a fever. I picked up a sixer, I've got *Sunday Night Football* on, the kid is doing his homework. I'm crushing it. I'm making the fuck out of this costume. I felt like I was... the guy. Who is that guy? The one from the show you watch?"

"Which one?"

"He wears those suits and is very proper. He designs clothes. Ted something?"

"Tim Gunn."

"I'm fucking Tim fucking Gunn, man. I used a portable sewing machine that Gladys sold me on. Under thirty dollars and surprisingly easy to use! I cut out white triangles for teeth. I bought huge googly eyes, which I hot-glued to the hood. The fabric was green and glittery. I taped some invisible streamers on the back for seaweed. At the end of the day, he looked fucking fantastic."

He pulled out his phone and showed her a picture of their adorable son, draped in glittered fabric with white triangles surrounding his face. Levi made a face to match the vile creature he thought he was.

"I thought it turned out pretty badass," said Shawn, proudly.

"It did," said Steph, smiling outwardly and inwardly.

They sat in silence, Shawn now anchored in her world, sitting in its cold air. The obdurate force that refused to yield to time, resting in its belief that it was helping to keep things the way they are: alive and well.

"You know, if Josh does wake up," he said. "And we do decide to take him. That would mean you and I are back together."

"Right."

"That leads me to something else I wanted to say. I moved back into the house. I just figured it would be-"

"Okay."

"And look, I'm really sorry. I know exactly what you meant. I was being a dick. Or, I mean, I get what you were saying. I get it, and I'm sorry. You're just too important, Steph, and so is Levi. I'm sorry. And I love you."

She pat him on the shoulder, smiling at him weakly. She rested her head there in a moment of quiet forgiveness. Her hand fell between them, swaying in the middle of the chasm between their chairs, Shawn's hand dangling as well. Their hands brushed together and then laced, finger through finger. Shawn held her hand firmly. Steph had forgotten how comforting he could be. She squeezed it hard in return, the rain and lightning strikes pounding the windows behind them.

"Oh," he said. He reached into the bag of dessert he had brought her. He removed the package of strawberry cheese-cake, cutting off a piece with a plastic fork. She took a bite, mulling over the taste.

"This is unbelievably bland," she said.

"Yeah," he said. "Well, at least they do something unbe-lievably well."

CHAPTER NINETEEN

JOSH STUMBLED OUT OF THE WOODS, GASPING AND walleyed. His tired legs tripped and sputtered like that of a torpid quarter horse, having spent its sprightly energy on a hopeless trek through a sprawling, unforgiving terrain. His lungs quavered as they sought the entirety of his realm's atmosphere, ballooning to an impossible extent. He fell to his knees in a brief moment of surrender, but a stabbing swivet reminded him in flashes of the fever dream he had just left, and he became alert again. Lightning illuminated the field before him, yawing grass visible in bursts of luminous, pale white. He felt the thunder through the ground, its palpable push scaring him back upon his tired, tremulous limbs. He raced forward several steps but turned to look back in curiosity. The woods remained, peering back with its thick forest of immovable darkness. Although he could not see or hear them, he felt the eyes of zombies. Their decrepit mitts stirring the air as they beckoned him back.

The rain intensified, building with Josh's increasing speed as he tore through the meadow. His legs sliced through the curling grass until he reached pavement, a surface he didn't know he had missed so dearly. The thunder persisted, along with the lightning that visibly struck the ground in the distance. It snapped into neighboring streets with the acrimonious blows akin to a reproachful slap on the knuckles by a bitter school nun. He kept running, dedicated to a destination he knew not of.

As he ran through the streets, he found them to be much more crowded than he left them. The familiar had returned, but they were in a doleful state. They resembled the dejected sight of his third-grade teacher, Mr. Flynn. They shuffled through the rainy streets, adorning soiled bed sheets and burlap blankets. Shanty towns populated the sidewalks with wind-beaten tents, rain damaged tarps and penurious wanderers without shelter who had no choice but to gather under the torn awnings of closed businesses. The faces that had once held warm grins of welcome now wore crooked smiles with ghoulish masks. Their hollowed eyes were filled with desperation and suspicion of one another. As he ran by them, they either whispered his name or cowered in fear of his quickness and capability. Rats scoured at their feet, gnawing on the ends of their ragged cloaks. Many of the vermin refused to move for Josh, instead, scuttling between his striding legs, clawing at his passing shoelaces.

The buildings had grown dark. Many of them were boarded up, showing no signs of denizens or that they had ever housed inhabitants. They were totemic relics in disrepair, emulous to the beleaguered masses who had gathered at their feet like stubborn acolytes to the statues of dead gods. Other than the intermittent strobe-like flash of lightning, the only light that managed to gleam in the vicinity of Josh was the Sears Tower, which still shone like the beacon it was, it's luminous beam hoisted high into the gloomy sky.

Josh ran towards it, through the increasing rain and the extended fingers of the deprived as they brushed at his passing ankles and hands. He approached the building and found a large encampment stationed just outside. A maze of tents and makeshift forts had inimically positioned themselves just outside, forcing him to hurriedly wander through sinuous paths of blowing fabric, inside which the defeated faces of his friends, teachers, babysitters, and neighborhood clerks squinted. Their beady eyes leered at him from their frigid, frail forts. Josh was torn. Should he stop? Could he help them? He was confused, not only by his gnawing morality but by the maze of fortresses that kept him from the front door. He had tried every which way, the dirtied faces encroaching with desperate pleas, the rain ossifying into a vigorous, cleaving fist, his exhaustion slowing his feet to a stammering wend. It wasn't until he had almost given up that he found the revolving door to the building.

He entered the lobby and was surprised to find it dark. The lights attempted to sputter to life like that of a rocking hull in the depths of a great ship, barreling through a torrential storm. It mimicked the vicious lightning strikes, fluttering to vibrant life, only to vanish again to darkness. Through the spastic illumination, he could just make out a figure standing by the elevator. It was Andy. He stood like a proper doorman. It was an eery sight, the lights flickering to reveal the smiling child standing alone. But regardless, Josh was relieved to see him.

"Hey, Joshy," said Andy. "Been waiting for ya. We got a big meeting to get to."

"It's bad out there, man."

"What do you mean?"

"All of those people? Did you see them?"

"Oh yeah. The bums. Forget them, man. We have more important things to tend to."

They entered the elevator, which had significantly aged, emulating the elevators from bygone eras. Andy pushed the button for their floor, and Josh cowered as the elevator jolted to life. He then performed a double-take when he noticed Andy's clothes: they were singed a charcoal black in fragmented patches as if they had been pulled from a fireplace. His skin was an unhealthy red; a violent sunburn covering his entire body.

"Andy. Are you okay?"

"Right as rain, partner. Right as rain," whispered Andy with a growing grin.

The elevator doors opened to reveal a dimly lit office. The cubicles were in disarray, some of their walls having been knocked down. Computers were turned over or unplugged, cabinets rifled through with files removed or thrown, desks were tossed and out of place. It looked as if there had been a last minute evacuation, his co-workers having left in a panic. Only Big Boy Bear remained. He stood in the center of the office, mixing the contents of a shaker and pouring them into a cocktail glass.

"Want a lil' sumfin to wet your whissle, Josshh? Zis meeting is gunna be a bitsh," said Big Boy, his voice greatly slurred.

Big Boy was supremely wasted, unable to bring his stitched mouth to his spilling drink. The rips in his sides had grown, the stains broadening to the size of continents on his matted fur. He tilted his head back and allowed what remained of the cocktail to pour onto his face. His drunk visage peering skyward, he lost his balance and tumbled backward over a cubicle wall. He landed with a soft thud, listless as he sat in the dread-filled silence. The atmosphere had become infected and diseased.

A phone rang. Josh's ears perked up, searching for the tocsin source. He looked to ask Andy, but he was no longer there. It rang again. He recognized the ring, the old bell ring of an old-fashioned rotary phone, but more specifically it was his grandmother's. It cut through the air with welcomed normalcy; a tone that told him all could be well again.

"Joshy. Let's go," said Andy, now appearing in the hall-way. He stood by the conference room door. "The meeting. You're gonna be late."

"Yeah. Hold on," he said. It rang and rang.

"Joshy. Now. Everyone is in here. They're waiting for you."

"Okay, but... I just feel like I gotta take this call."

"Don't take it, Joshy."

"I'm sorry, but..." He searched and searched. He was closer. "Hold on, Andy."

He found the phone, which rested on his desk. His was the only cubicle in pristine condition, looking completely undisturbed. His prescient beliefs were predicated as it was indeed his grandmother's black rotary phone. It used to sit in her kitchen. The same one she would let ring and ring, saying, "Let it be. It's just the bill collectors." It rang again. Josh felt its magnetism and reached for it, lifting the receiver to his ear.

"Are you ready?" asked the voice.

"Is this you? Or, I mean, is this the woman? From the alley?"

"Are you ready?" she asked again, persistent and in the same tone.

Josh was flustered. He looked for Andy and Big Boy, but

they were nowhere to be found. How could he answer such an impossible question?

"I don't know," he said. "I don't know what to do. I don't think I should leave my friends. I think they need me."

"Everything has changed, hasn't it?"

"Yes. It's terrible."

"Right. So, you should leave."

"Yeah..." he said, still uncertain. "I know I should."

"It's going to get worse."

"Are you sure?"

"I am."

"How do you know?"

"Don't I sound like I know?"

"...yeah..."

"Okay, then. Let's go."

"But I still have friends here."

"No. You don't."

"I do. I'm looking at one of them right now," he said, looking at Andy who had appeared again by the door of the conference room. Andy motioned to his tiny calculator watch, signifying they were running late.

"I'm sorry, but I have a meeting to go to," said Josh.

"So you're saying no? You're not ready yet? Is that correct?"

"Let's say, hypothetically of course, that I did say no to whatever it is you're trying to get me to say yes to. What would happen?"

She sighed with eternal regret.

"You all try to stay. You grasp to the holograms of your memory only because they're known, but they provide no sustenance. People like to remember things. There is no fault in that. But the folly lies in time and intent. There is nothing worth meaning here, Joshua. You can only recycle the physical and mental so many times until its fabric wears thin and finally dissolves to nothingness. It is people like you, Joshua, who fail to realize that some things are meant to be forgotten."

Josh sat on the phone, trying to dissect the woman's upbraiding. He looked to Andy who waved him over, emphatically now. Sensing Josh's trepidation, she sighed again, heavily.

"It's going to become more difficult for you, Josh. If you don't come now, it will become very, very difficult."

"Okay, well..." he said, not knowing what was going to come next. He looked to Andy and then back to the phone. "Like I said, I have this meeting I have to go to. They're all sort of waiting on me? So, I'm going to hop in real quick, just for a sec, and then I'll come right back. So maybe call back in like..." he pulled his face away, covering the receiver with his hand. "Is twenty minutes good, Andy? Fifteen, maybe? How long we thinking?" he called to his friend.

"This shouldn't take long, Joshy," said Andy.

Josh gave Andy a thumbs up and returned to the phone. "Yeah, let's make it fifteen. Call me back in fifteen. Cool?"

"So it's a no," she said, flatly.

"It's a 'not right now, but in fifteen minutes.' Also, I have a couple more questions. Where-"

The building shook, the ground rolling underneath him. The remaining cubicle walls fell in unison like tumbling playing cards. The desks and chairs rattled. Josh felt the entire building sway. The lights went dark, the only light now coming from the gloomy color of the storm raging beyond the office windows. Josh looked around in such hysterics that he almost missed the woman's voice through the phone. She was repeating a phrase, over and over again. He pressed his ear to the phone.

"Get out and get home," she said.

"Miss!" he screamed. "Something is happening here!"

"Get out," she said. "And get home. Get out and get home."

The line went dead. His desk bounced across the floor, ripping the phone cord from the floor and carrying it with it.

"Andy?!" cried Josh. He looked around for his friend, but he was nowhere to be seen. "Andy, where are you? Big Boy?"

Josh tripped over loose wires and fallen office furniture. He scrambled toward the windows to look out onto the city. He pressed his palms against them, stabilizing himself, and staring out into the storm. The squall ravaged the city with its pale green clouds, the gusts of wind-shattering windows and causing the buildings to sway like Jenga towers. The infrastructure had crumbled, causing the parlous streets to flood with rivulets of wild rainwater. The camps that had formed in front of the buildings were swept away, their temporary owners scattering like discovered cockroaches.

The Empire State Building wavered, its windows bursting and chunks of masonry becoming dislodged, hurtling towards the ground. It looked as if it were made of sugar, slowly dissolving in the rain. The left side of the building broke free, crumbling to the flooded avenues. It fell like an anguished hand, clutching to what was left and bringing the rest down with it. The surrounding buildings caught fire, smoke pluming from their windows. The billows fused with the opaque fog that had now slid between the buildings like hungry tendrils, clutching to structures in the hopes of strangling the life from them. They fell in fire and smoke and rain, their ruinous fate signifying the perished verisimilitude of Josh's once bountiful surroundings of comfort and optimism. The biblical disaster unfolded with rapacious hunger, a primal want for everything he had ever held dear to him. It vowed to take.

"Come on, Joshy. Let's go."

Josh found Andy at the end of the hall. He stood, smoldering. Obsidian smoke rose from his pulsating skin. He radiated with enormous heat, his body breaking apart and his skin bubbling with hideous scars. His scorched eyes were coal black, and he flashed a wolfish grin, allowing a miasma of iniquity to fume from his maw and seep into the space.

"Andy?" whimpered Josh.

With a burst of fire Andy's eyes flared to life. They flickered with licking flames, searing into Josh's fearful gaze with the prophetic confidence of what was to come. Josh stood enraptured by his friend's burning image. All sound was drowned out as a whirlpool of confusion engulfed him, and the windows of the building burst and his friend became a ball of flames.

CHAPTER TWENTY

I ASKED SHAWN TO TAKE LEVI HOME. OUR BOY HAS BEEN such a trooper, desperately wanting to be there for his mom. But I can tell that this environment, this entire situation, has been wearing on him. Or, maybe that's just me projecting. But every time I look at him, he flashes me a smile. He just wants to help me, anyway that he can.

Mom and Dad just left. Mom complained that her blood sugar was crashing, and Dad kept repeating the phrase, "I think a good, eight hours will do me just right." Although both of these complaints were voiced after I brought up the paperwork and the decision of whether or not to sign it. I made sure that my ambivalence to their presence was properly communicated, and was happy to watch them leave.

It's up to me, I keep telling myself. If I don't figure this out, no one will. Only I can fix this. They need to go home because I need to save them. I feel the delusion in my brain festering like a tumor.

I'm in the room by myself again, which is how I prefer it. People have oscillated back and forth, coming and going, but

Josh and my presence remains the constant. That and the water damage. I believe there is a leak somewhere in the ceiling. The brown stain above us has gradually grown over the course of the two weeks that we've been here. It feels like a looming cloud, gathering size as it threatens to storm. No one has made mention of it, which I find very odd as I cannot help but track its movement. With everyone's blithe dismissal, it begins to feel like an imaginary friend. I want to interact with it, make silly faces at it, perform for it. I don't know. I'm tired. Also, did I mention that I am supremely bored? I am. Very, very bored. I have Josh, my imaginary friend, and my window that looks out onto the lawn and the McDonalds across the street. Sometimes I literally watch the grass grow.

More accurately, I have been watching hair grow. Having run a gauntlet of physical terror, Josh looks unrecognizable to me. His face is bruised and swollen. Tubes invade him like thirsty leeches, pumping liquids in and obviating the toxic waste from his stiff body. I bought a hairbrush at the Walgreens nearby, along with some other hygiene products. I imagine if he were aware right now that he would want to look, and smell, somewhat presentable.

Josh was due for a haircut by the time of the accident, and with part of his head shaved for the operation, he looks like a deranged punk rocker. If I were able to tell him this, he would laugh. His facial hair has fuzzed forth, although he hasn't been here long enough to resemble a caveman. He could never grow that kind of beard even if he were given two years, let alone two weeks. The beard currently crowding his mug is patchy and sharp. An abomination of beards, similar to the time he tried to grow a mustache. He had just left for college, a freshman, so he had only been gone for a total of like, three months when he came home for Christmas. The sight of my brother sauntering to the front door, a thin layer of dirt above his lip, sent my mother into shamed appall. She made him shave it.

"You look like you sell smut," she said.

My Dad still brings that one up.

The state of Josh's current beard is so offensive that I am determined to mend it. I bought a razor and some shaving cream at the drug store. If I'm going to be alone with him, then he has to at least look like some version of the brother I grew up with.

Maybe, in a few years, he could have grown himself a good beard. It took Dad until his early forties to grow an excellent beard, but he could always nail the mustache. When he was in the service, when we were just kids, he always had a mustache. He shaved it one time without telling us. He showed up at my school to pick me up, and I was so terrified by the physical change that I refused to get in the car.

"That man is not my father!" I screamed.

Josh surely would have attempted to grow a mustache, to be just like Dad; probably when he got into his forties. We'd all remark that he "looks just like him!" But waiting so long to grow it, he'd be disappointed to find that it would only grow with streaks of grey.

"Should I dye it?" you'd ask me.

"No. Please don't," I'd say. "You'll look like one of those guys who hang out downtown, trying to lure college girls into their Camaro."

And maybe, by that time, you would have dumped that god-awful Raina. What the fuck were you thinking? That had absolutely zero legs. You'd be with someone much more kind; someone intellectually stimulating. You would be through with your "I wanna be with hot girls" phase, and you would have decided to settle down with someone nerdy. Sure, I would be standoffish at first, but it would just be my insecurity. Once I realized how funny she was, and how she liked to give you a hard time like I do, I'd decide that you were perfect for each other. But then you'd do something crazy, like go off and get married without telling anyone. And you'd come to me first, before Mom and Dad.

"What were you thinking?" I'd say.

"We weren't thinking. That's the point!" you'd say, very excited as usual.

"Look, I love her," I'd say. "But you've only been dating a year. Shawn and I were together for four before we made the jump. Are you sure this was the smart move?"

"I don't know," you'd say. "All I know is it feels right. Right now, it feels right. I love her, and I want to be with her. That should be enough."

And there would be nothing I could say to that. You'd agree that at least you want to make it appear as if you hadn't gotten married yet. So, you'd decide to fake an engagement in front of Mom and Dad. They'd go ballistic, so happy for you. And you have your wedding. Of course, even though it's basically a sham, it's the best wedding I've ever been to. There's tons of stupid dancing and fantastic food. Mom would be so happy because you'd appease her by doing the ceremony at the Evanston parish. You'd do that mother-son dance to something overly sentimental like *"You Raise Me Up"* by Josh Groban. It would be so disgusting and lame, but Mom would be crying tears of exultant joy. Dad would get drunk and would keep telling you how proud he is of you. And you'd make everyone do the fucking chicken dance. I'd hate it, but of course, you'd know that. That's why you chose it: to piss me off and force me to do something I don't want to do. The whole wedding would be so embarrassing and corny and over-the-top and somehow weirdly awesome. Just like everything you ever did.

As I'm putting the shaving cream on your face, I realize that I don't know how to do this. Is shaving a face different from shaving a leg? You move downward, for sure, but do you shave up? What if I cut you? As I smooth out the lather, I realize that I've put too much on. It's a thick icing on your round face. You look like a demented cupcake. You would have laughed at that. Not to mention, the razor is legitimately terrible. Guy razors are so weird. Why do they have to make them so different? It keeps pulling on the hair in the same way Dad used to complain about. Do you remember that?

"The God damn thing is tugging at my face like it's mad at me!" he'd yell.

"Rich! Don't use his name in vain!" Mom would yell back.

"Buy me something other than these damn disposables, and I'll get down on bended knee, Lisa!"

I would be wrong, by the way, about you rushing to get married. It would work out, of course. You guys would be so great together. I imagine that your wife would be a teacher. Like, first grade. She has an expansive imagination, just like yours. And you guys would nerd out over everything together; all the things you love: *Star Wars*, comic books, superhero movies. Uch. Fucking nerds. Then, she'd get pregnant. I'd be shocked, so of course, I'd be really annoying and say things like, "Are you sure you guys are ready for this?" and "It's a lot of responsibility, Josh," and "It's not all fun and games."

I wouldn't be able to conceptualize you as a father. No offense, but even though you're older, I've always felt like the older sibling. But then you'd have a boy. He'd be blond like you were when you were a kid. And he'd have your imagination, but he'd be sneaky like I was. "Crafty," Mom always said. And oh my god Mom would lose her fucking mind over this kid because he would look so much like you. She'd be over at your house, constantly. She'd just obsess over him. I'd get jealous and bitter, feeling like she was neglecting Levi. She loves Levi, but she has always been waiting for a grandbaby from you. I'd confront her about it, but she would, of course, deny it. You were always the favorite, and whenever I brought that to her attention, she would either harangue me with a heated lecture or roll her eyes and scoff. But I wouldn't be jealous for long because your boy would be so sweet, just like you. And even though he and Levi would be apart in age, they'd still get along. And I could finally be there for you. You'd have all sorts of questions:

"What's the right diaper brand?"

"Should he sleep on his tummy or his back?"

"We're too busy to breastfeed. What do we do?!"

I'd answer all of your questions. I'd finally be there to help you. Not that you would need it. You would grow in your career, finally getting some bigger position at your company. You'd be a lauded designer in your field, traveling for conferences in the summer so your wife could come. We'd watch the boy while you were away. But then you'd move into management, stop working so much on the ground floor of things.

"Wow, I'm surprised you made such a responsible move," I'd say. "Sometimes it's good to make a decision based around money, huh?"

But then you'd say, "I'm actually more excited about the opportunity to manage other programmers. I want to mentor and watch other people flourish."

And that would bug the hell out of me because I would

wonder how it was that you always had an answer for everything.

The human neck has so many divots and slopes. The hair moves in so many directions, it's impossible to tell if I'm shaving down or up. I'm washing the razor in a bowl by your bed, and it's getting water and foam everywhere. I've made a terrible mess.

We'd get old. Mom would go, as she seems to be threatening more and more lately. Dad, too. It would be hard to watch, but we'd have each other. It would end up bringing us closer. We'd be closer than we ever thought possible. And now with Levi off and married, and your son going off to college, we could start traveling together. We'd go to Europe, Southeast Asia, the Caribbean. We'd love Hawaii, so much so that we'd decide to go halves on a condo. And we'd fight over it; who gets it during the colder months. You'd let me win, which I would know and resent. You'd be doing so well that you'd do something like get another vacation place, except it would be in the woods. The opposite. I'd be sitting on a beach in the winter time, jealous that you're in the mountains somewhere, bundled up in the cold.

"You've always been jealous," you'd say.

I wipe off your face. Not bad.

"You nicked me here and there, but overall I agree," you'd say. "Not bad. Way to go, Sis!"

"Don't mock me," I'd say.

"I'm not mocking you," you'd say. "I'm being genuine. Way to go!"

"What should I do?" I'd ask you if I could.

"I can't tell you that," you'd say. "You've always known what to do. You've held that over my head my entire life."

"But now I'm not so sure," I'd say.

"You want me to tell you? Is my little sister actually asking for my advice?" you'd say.

"Yes! Okay? Yes! Please tell me," I'd say.

"I think you need to give me permission," you'd say.

"I can't do that," I'd say. "I can't give you permission."

"You have more ahead of you," you'd say. "People who need you. But I don't need you. Give me permission."

"I wouldn't be able to forgive myself," I'd say.

"That's dumb," you'd say. "This wasn't your fault."

"But then what happens to you?" I'd ask.

"I don't know," you'd say. "But wherever it is, it's where everyone else is hanging out. And I'll just be there, and one day you'll show up. Or maybe you won't, Steph. Maybe you'll go to hell."

"Josh!" I'd say.

"I'm just saying! There are no guarantees," you'd say. "I can try to work my magic and put in a good word, but don't hold your breath. Just try not to become Jeffrey Dahmer while you're alive and you're probably fine."

"You're such an asshole," I'd say.

He would see that I was emotional and he would get awkward because that's what he always did.

"Are you sure?" I'd ask.

"Yeah. I am," he'd say.

"But, Josh. I need you to be you," I'd say.

"I need you to tell me," he'd say. "So do it, Steph. Go ahead. Ready?"

"No," I'd say.

"What do you need from me?" he'd ask, expectantly.

I'd hesitate, but I'd gather some courage.

"Go. I need you to go," I'd finally say.

"Thanks, Sis," he'd say. "That means a lot."

I reach into my purse where I've stashed some of Dad's

aftershave. I stole it, figuring my brother would like to smell like him. He used the old stuff, the brand that made the talcum powder that every barbershop used. I poured a puddle in my hand, probably too much, and slapped it on.

"Yowza!" you'd say. Just like Dad, every time.

What a funny, weird thing to do.

CHAPTER TWENTY-ONE

THE OFFICE WAS SUBMERGED WITHIN THE STRANGLING thickness of black, poisonous smoke. The fire had spread throughout the building, its enraged flames snaking their way through the office with eager voracity. Although he could not see him, Josh felt the heat of his childhood friend somewhere amongst the stygian clouds. The menacing warmth had intensified, scalding his skin to a fearful degree. He couldn't breathe, his lungs feeling dry and shrunken. His escalated body heat made him ill and queasy. As both his internal and external temperature surged, he knew Andy was growing closer.

A ball of erratic flames became visible, spastically whorling amongst the smoke like a small star in space. The flames frenetically popped and leaped into the air, only to return to the lumbering mass. The small sun had built a gravitational pull, gathering objects closer, which included Josh, who was sliding, against his will, towards the flaming maw. He stopped himself, gasping to an office corner. The star inched closer.

Josh, on hands and knees, crawled in the opposite direction. He shuffled, staring at his hands as they scrambled over scorched desk items. There were pictures of Pat Perlola, Lou Fetherman, and Leia Foth. The bodies were decrepit and mummified, the frames burnt, and the pictures bubbling. Lumps of carpet peeled like scar tissue, curling and singeing as it removed itself from the office floor.

In a persistent crawl, Josh finally hit the crown of his head on the elevator door. He rose quickly, pushing the button for escape. But the doors refused to open. He searched for the stairs, a fire escape, anything. There was nothing. The heat had escalated to a hellish degree, the fire now consuming the office in its entirety. The ball of swirling flames plodded towards him, now with outstretched arms, a demonic countenance finding its way through the blaze and staring into Josh's terrified expression. His back to the wall, Josh closed his eyes in capitulation to the superior, galactic force. The heat grew and grew.

The walls behind him opened and Josh fell backward. As the elevator doors closed, he could just make out Andy's grim, fiery figure as he reached for him. The old elevator jolted to life and shot downwards like a brick dropped from a bridge. He hurtled towards the ground at a reckless speed, the falling box roasting like an oven as it hurtled towards earth.

As he reached the lobby, the doors didn't open so much as they fell off. Josh dashed forward but was surprised to find himself enveloped in damp, molding fluff. He stood, dazed, as he realized the pillowy mold filled the entirety of the lobby, stacked to his waste. It reeked of dried booze and garden compost. He waded through the stuffing of his childhood bear as it squirmed around him, gripping at his trudging legs like hungry quicksand. It was a pool of palms without fingers, squeezing and grasping at Josh's limbs as he struggled to grind forward. Bits of quivering hide rippled on top of the frothy mass. As he bound forward, Josh spotted watchful button eyes, peering as he passed. Loose stitching snaked through the ocean of brownish-grey like angry sea snakes. The fluff closed around his extremities, hugging his waist like a mother begging her son not to enlist. Josh kicked and scratched as he made his way through the tremulous, fluffy intestines, towards the revolving door, and into the waiting storm.

He fell through the revolving doors and onto the wet side-walk where the rain attacked him from a sideways slant. It was a wall of storm, the sky unleashing upon him. It battered Josh with wind and water, thunder howling as lightning flashed.

"Josh," said a reed the voice, lazily falling through the heavy downpour.

Keira came towards him, stumbling with tenuous, plod-ding steps. Needles protruded from every inch of her skin, jagged and rusty as they pierced the air around her like a dead porcupine. Her skin was yellow and blanched. As she opened her mouth, a viscous ectoplasm rolled forth, slopping down her chin. Her eyes were empty shells of white, wide in horrific ecstasy.

"You'll always be my guy, Josh," she said with a duplici-tous gargle.

The Sears Tower shook, along with the buildings beside it. They quaked and rattled, bumping into one another. Loose detritus fell, smashing into the ground around him. The tower shook, and all at once, every window burst. The obsidian shards mixed with the rain and fell with brute, ruinous force. Josh ducked, covering his head as if he were hiding under his desk during a 1950's bomb scare. The shards of plummeting knives slashed his skin, slicing open his shoulders, back, and neck. The blood ran down his down-turned face, dripping onto the flooded pavement, pooling and running away with the passing streams.

"Joshy!" cried Andy.

He exited the revolving doors of the Sears Tower, the fiery figure sauntering towards Josh. The fluff behind him burned like a torched field of wheat. The flames quickly climbed the once eminent building, now a massive, blazing structure filling the sky with fire and smoke.

Josh's Coupe Deville sat on blocks, ravaged and immovable. He frantically searched, but there were no other vehicles on the streets.

He found his childhood bike chained to a mailbox on the corner, just as he used to do in the front of his middle school. It was a five-speed mountain bike with a rattling chain and weak brakes that his father had bought him at a garage sale. He scurried towards it, pulling at the chain, but found it restricted by his old combination lock. He whirled the knob forwards, backward, and forwards again until the correct combination came to him. The lock popped off, and he hopped on his old bike. The rusted chain sputtered as it searched for traction amongst the damaged gears. His pedaling was labored and impaired by his damaged muscles and smoke-filled lungs. As he came off the curb, the front tire landed in a sewer grate and launched him over the front handlebars. He hit the street with a harsh thud, his shoulder slamming into its socket.

He winced, rolling on his back, the rain unforgivably stabbing into his face like the glass of the building before. His burning friend crawled towards him from the corner of his eye. Rats emerged from the sewer, climbing atop Josh's bleeding body, gnawing at his open wounds. Josh cried and shook them off, stumbling to his feet. He propped himself unsteadily back on his bike. As he pedaled, he felt that both tires were flat. The metal frames ground into the street, allowing him to feel every stone and pebble in his stiff, bloody wrists and palms. He bounced, his teeth rattling as his legs forced every downward push. As he increased his speed, he turned to see the Sears Tower fall, a pillar of ash crumbling to the ground, bringing the remaining buildings with it.

He followed an unspoken sense as he pedaled toward an unknown destination. His legs were empty of blood and oxygen, his clothes ragged and torn. His arms bled from the lacerations, the sticky red congealing between his fingers as they gripped the rubber handlebars. He zigged and zagged through the fractured asphalt, careening over vast upheavals and dangerous potholes.

He finally saw it: the neighborhood. He coasted through the rotting houses of old neighbors and television families. The roofs had caved, and moss had laid siege to the exteriors of the old stalwarts. He found his home, ditching the bike on the front lawn as he had done so many times before. He stopped on the front porch and glanced back at the city. It was an inky cloud of smoke and fury, flickers of blaze managing to rage against the torrential downpour. The flames had reached beyond the city limits, forcing a clear path towards the neighborhood. The glowing ball was conducting the pursuit, approaching in the distance like the leader of a gang of ominous outlaws.

Josh dashed inside the home, searching for any indication that this was where he was supposed to be. But all he found was rot and decay. The wizened house had been gutted, walls knocked down, furniture and familiar knick-knacks pilfered. An odious, acrid mold climbed the walls; a malcontent fungus. Water trickled from the ceiling like a Medieval dungeon. He could hear the guts of the home fracturing, tearing. The stitching of the memories that had been impetuously sewn together were violently ripping themselves from one another like curdling milk. Josh asked himself why he was where he was, but there was no answer. It was a last-ditch hope.

He returned to the street, staring fondly at the diseased house as it fell, room-by-room. Andy slogged down the road, fire behind him. As he passed, homes erupted in flames and crumbled to ash.

"Joshua," said the woman in black.

She stood on his childhood lawn, her hand outstretched. She wore a worried look, shaking her hand with urgency.

"Are you ready?" she asked.

Whispering, but not from her. Josh searched for the source of the rustling. He found another woman behind him. This one he knew recognized, but couldn't quite place. Josh struggled to hear her through the rain. He tried to reach her, scrambling towards her, but the storm intensified, making her impossible to reach. He was positive he knew her. She looked despondent, but her jaw kept moving, speaking directly to him. It pained him that he couldn't hear.

"Hello!" he cried. "Excuse me! What are you saying?"

"Joshua," said the woman in black, standing impatiently on the lawn.

"No, I'm sorry. Hold on, she's trying to say something!"

The figure he recognized, but did not yet know, kept speaking, only barely decipherable. He fought against the onslaught of wind, inching closer.

"What do you want me to do?" he barely heard her squeak.

Josh was dumbfounded.

"I don't know! I... I'm not sure I can tell you that." He waited for a reply.

"But now I'm not so sure," he heard her say, hardly being able to make it out.

"Joshua," said the woman in black. "We need to go."

His recognition grew. He knew her more than anyone he had met in this place. It was the first emotional warmth he had felt since he could remember. He couldn't leave her.

"Please! Tell me what to do!" she boomed, suddenly crystal clear. Josh was startled, pushed to his heels.

"I mean it, Joshua," said the woman in black. "Now."

Andy crept closer, the wall of flames behind him. They had reached the neighboring house.

"I think I have to go," said Josh to the woman he knew he loved. "Is that okay? I'm sorry, but I think I have to."

"But then what happens to you?" she asked him.

"I don't know."

"Are you sure?"

Andy was here with resonant fury. The woman in black reached her hand out again.

"Yeah," said Josh. "I am."

"But I need you."

Josh was broken by the crestfallen face. It impacted him so profoundly that it only cemented how much he cared for her.

"I don't want to leave you, but I have to," said Josh. "Is that okay? I'm so sorry, but I have to go. Can I? Can I go? Do I have your permission to go?"

She hesitated, but he saw her gather courage.

"Go. I need you to go."

"Thank you. That means a lot. I hope to see you again."

"Joshua!" cried the woman in black.

He took this as his final cue and ran for the woman in black, but just before he grabbed her hand, he heard a phrase he had not heard in years. Through the wind and the rain and the raging fire, he heard her say, "Yowza!" It was her. It was Steph. He turned, but the elements were fiercely insuperable. He wanted to reach her. Andy was close. The heat was intense. The last thing Josh ever felt was the touch of a woman's hand whom he did not know.

CHAPTER TWENTY-TWO

THE TABLE OF SNACKS THAT LISA AND STEPH HAD prepared were in the theme of Josh's favorites. For appetizers, there were Lisa's deviled eggs, which he and Rich were known to devour in late-evenings/early-mornings of holidays. Along with a hearty potato salad (decidedly anti-gourmet, i.e., the kind that tasted like it belonged in tupperware containers for picnics by a lake). For the main course, they had hired a small, local caterer (Steph's doing, much to her mother's chagrin) who had prepared lamb skewers and turkey tacos (extra guacamole), as well as gourmet chili dogs, which was the chef's take on a dish that Rich used to make the kids when Lisa was away for the weekend ("shit on a shingle" is what he called it). Then came the desserts, which were always Josh's favorite. His mother made her famous caramel popcorn balls, which were just buttered popcorn mixed with melted caramel, shaped into ball-form, and with a finishing dash of salt. Steph had purchased a Halloween-sized bag of Butterfingers, which she had cut up and piled together to create a mountainous "cake." And there was

French Vanilla ice cream, which was somehow Josh's favorite flavor of ice cream.

As to be expected, the funeral had been taxing, but what Steph did not expect was to find some relief within it. It served as a peculiar form of punctuation to the draining ordeal. They had been mourning Josh from the moment he entered the hospital, and while the wake was more of an opportunity for others to grieve, she felt that it bookended their tragedy rather nicely. She had slept well the previous night, something she had not expected. Maybe that was because she was sharing a bed with Shawn again; she always slept better with him there, even though he was a notorious bed hog. Levi had been in a surprisingly good mood this morning. He made Steph and Shawn laugh with a dirty joke that he learned from a friend at school, which he didn't know was dirty.

Overall, she felt strangely lighthearted. Perhaps it was the wine. She had downed several glasses of the dark Bordeaux she had brought and hidden in the kitchen. Even in Lisa's deepest mourning, she still kept a watchful eye on how much alcohol Steph consumed, offering minatory, sideways glances and mental tallying. Steph sat in the high-backed reading chair in the corner, observing people as they interacted. She imagined that she was Josh, an apparition, watching people talk about him. She was amused by the odd pairings of strangers. Most of them had no business speaking with one another.

"And how did you know Josh?"

"So, you're from here? Or did you say you moved?"

"And remind me again, what do you do for work?"

"I'm sorry, I don't think I got your name. Was it Stanley? Or Steven?"

This was the most fun she had had in weeks. She

polished off her glass and stood, eager to replete her resources. She felt a slight bend in her knees and a subtle sway. She had to slow down, or things could get out of hand. The last thing Steph wanted was to make the scene that everyone thought was possible. She had already spilled on her black skirt; her "outfit of sorrow" was actually just an all-black work outfit that she commonly wore Monday through Friday; she had several like it. She had spilled on it many times after coming home from a stressful day and popping a bottle. It did an excellent job of either ridding itself of stains or masking them from the human eye.

"Stephanie?" asked a man with the look of a town butcher. He was bulbous and balding, his meaty paws looking like catcher's mitts. He had a hefty gut and was red in the face, tantamount to a toddler who had just stifled a crying fit.

"You probably don't recognize me, do you?" he said.

"Of course I do," she said with drunken duplicity. "You were friends with Josh."

This was, of course, an audacious guess. But Steph was in a state of irreverence and willing to give into cavalier impulses.

"Well, 'friends' may be a little strong," said the man. "I kind of... jeez, this is embarrassing. I used to, kind of, bully Josh. In middle school. Some in high school, too. My name is Dewey Reese."

Stephanie lit up. The presence of a school bully excited her. She saw herself, throughout Josh's life, as somewhat of a bully to him. While perhaps not as brutal as Josh had reported Dewey Reese to be, she often liked to chip away at her brother with psychological, and sometimes physical, blows. He was fun to tease. She also knew Dewey for additional reasons: she had dated his younger brother, Travis, for a short, three-month period. They had been each other's dates for Spring Formal and had capped their romantic affair with a terrible, public make-out display in the middle of a matinee showing of *Star Wars, Episode II: Attack of the Clones.* She had gone over to Travis's house once to fool around in his bedroom when his father was drunk and unaware. She remembered seeing Dewey putting him to bed, his father falling over himself and slurring incoherently. She felt like an undercover agent, seeing another side of the infamous enemy.

"Ah yes, the famous Dewey Reese," she said.

"Yeah, I guess I sorta was," he said, grimly. "God, I just feel terrible about that stuff."

"Oh, don't. He was a very bully-able kid," she laughed. "You actually missed the 'Bully Wake.' It was a special wake we had just for Josh's bullies. Huge turnout. Packed to the rafters."

This made Dewey laugh and relax.

"I just wanted to say that I'm really sorry for your loss," said Dewey. "Josh was always a good guy. That's why I think I picked on him. I was jealous. When you guys moved here, he made friends immediately. Which bugged the living hell out of me. It was so hard for me to do that sort of thing. But everyone liked Josh. It all came so easy to him. Seeing someone be so care-free just makes you-"

"Makes you want to wring his neck. Look, like I said, I get it. Take it from one of his other bullies, I get it."

She saw Dewey grow short of breath, his eyes reddening and gathering mist.

"That's really nice to hear," he said, pitifully.

Steph grew sincere but also disappointed that Dewey was a much more somber presence than she was hoping for. She decided she needed more wine.

"Thank you for coming, Dewey," she said, putting a hand on his shoulder. "Make sure you grab some lamb skewers. The caterer is phenomenal. And tell your brother I said hi."

"He's living in Tulsa. Selling tires. He's very happy," he said, tears welling.

"That's great to hear."

He smiled, agreeing, and walked away. As he did, Steph's gaze turned to the living room where adults were seated with sallow faces. Standing in the middle of the room were Levi and his friends. Ever the popular little boy, he had amassed a group of jocular kids his age. Although Levi had always had a special connection with Josh, the weight of the moment was too large for him to comprehend. So instead, he held court in front of his friends, making fart noises on his forearm. He deployed the classic mouth-to-arm technique.

"That's the best way," said Levi, proudly displaying his false-flatulence technique.

"No, you gotta put your hand in your armpit and flap it like a chicken," said one of the boys. He showcased the move with loud, audible farts, making additional noises with his mouth for good measure. The boys giggled hysterically.

"I think the best way is when you blow into your elbow. Like this," said another boy. He demonstrated, which was the loudest of the mouth farts.

"Oh man!" cried Levi. "That was a juicy one!"

While this was wildly inappropriate, Steph couldn't help but laugh. The boys were surrounded by despondent adults, all glowering at the boisterous youths, frustrated by their impudence towards the idea of death and permanence. They looked like the audience of the Roman Coliseum, grimly staring at the indecorous display of mouth-fart violence between young gladiators. Steph thought it best to split it up, but just before she could, Shawn swooped in.

He gathered the boys carefully, rounding them up like cattle.

"Alright, boys. Let's fart outside, shall we?" he said, ushering them to the back door. Levi nodded to the other boys and led them dashing out the back.

Shawn caught Steph's eye and accompanying smile. He walked towards her, grabbing a Butterfinger on the way. He gave her a chocolate-covered kiss, peanut butter and chocolate clinging to her lips. She left it there for a moment before licking it off.

"How you doin'? More wine?" asked Shawn.

"I'm doing fine, and yes. I think I hid it in the kitchen."

"I know, but your mom found it. 'Whose is this? Well, whosever it is, it looks like they're having their way with it.' I relocated it to the sideboard."

Shawn shuffled, sneakily, to the sideboard next to them. He opened a hatch and brandished the half-drunk bottle of red. He filled her glass, then dramatically glanced over each shoulder like a vaudevillian comic, making sure no one was looking. He returned the bottle to its hiding place.

"Very nice," she said. "Speaking of, have you seen my mother?"

"Kitchen. Just so you know, I tried to stop her."

Steph knew the implied meaning and scoffed, rolling her eyes.

"Jesus," she said. "Oops. No god talk. My bad."

Steph crossed to the kitchen where she found Lisa scrubbing away at a mountain of dishes.

"Mom, no. Just wait until after and I'll do them. Some of these aren't even ours, they're the caterer's."

"I just want to make myself useful."

"This is why I said we should have done paper plates."

"My goodness, it's a wake, Stephanie. Not a Fourth of July barbecue."

"It's fine, Mom, just go out there and say hello to people. All of your friends are here."

"I cannot accept one more person's condolences. It's exhausting."

"Okay then, how about we go outside and get some fresh air?"

Lisa stopped scrubbing, removing her dish gloves and drying her hands on a towel by the stove. She stared for a moment, wondering if that was what she wanted.

"Okay," she said, finally.

As they walked out back, the heel on Steph's left shoe buckled momentarily, causing her to briefly lose her balance. She clung to her mother's shoulder, steadying herself.

"Oh no, Stephanie. You're not drunk are you?"

"Mom! No. I've had two glasses. It's these heels. I knew I should have worn flats."

Her mother gave her a dubious look but patted her still resting hand and continued outside. Steph was most certainly drunk, but happily. She was also surprised by the sturdiness of her mother's figure. It filled her with a glow of eternal happiness to know that she could still cling to her vital mother to keep herself from falling. She wasn't as weak as she previously thought.

Lisa and Steph came out onto the back deck where they found Shawn and Rich in the yard with the exiled boys. They had devised a confused game of tag that revolved around Shawn and Rich acting like zombified monsters. The boys ran between the garage and a large oak tree that, Steph guessed, were each serving as a home base. If the men managed to wrap the boys up, they were "infected," and would join the zombie army. Levi darted between the sluggish adults, screaming as he scurried from base to base. But, being distracted by his approaching grandfather, he didn't see his dad approaching from behind. Shawn captured him, holding onto his son as he squealed, lifting him high into the air.

Steph watched her mother with deep interest. She was smiling as she watched Rich lumber around the yard after the boys.

"No matter how old he gets, he will never be too old to act like a fool," said Lisa with a sideways smile.

Rich paused a moment, collecting his breath. His hands went to his knees as he sucked wind. A few of the boys gathered around him, feeling his lassitude and inevitable surrender. They knew the game could end at any moment with the famously uttered adult line, "Well, that's enough of that. I'm beat."

But Rich's exhaustion was merely a ploy; a sneaky tactic from the wily old man. He roared to life and clutched to one of the boys, enveloping him in a massive bear hug. The boy laughed, then slowly transformed, plodding across the lawn with Rich.

Steph was already out of wine. She estimated that if she had another glass that she will have indulged in three-quarters of a bottle. She suppressed the urge to venture inside to the sideboard. She decided instead to savor the moment in the backyard. She could feel it slipping through her fingers. The family was outside. It was a balmy, fall day. The kids were laughing. Mom was smiling. Dad was acting like a monster. Shawn was tossing Levi into the air.

But Rich finally grew winded, and Levi wished to be put down.

"Well, that's enough of that," said Rich. "I'm beat."

One by one, the adults filtered back inside. Steph

watched as Levi and his friends were thrust into a momentary state of creative paralysis. Steph smiled, nodding to her son encouragingly. She followed her mother back into the kitchen, leaving the children to come up with a new game to play.

ACKNOWLEDGMENTS

Thank you to my wife, Kate Cobb, for serving as both supporter and editor, pushing me to plan the future without dwelling too much in the past. Jeff Bigley for his recollection of people and places, and Jeanie Bigley's tolerance of incessant medical questions. Annie for long walks through writer's block. To Leza Cantoral and Christoph Paul at CLASH. Thank you to Laura Wilkinson for her ambitious push, Ryan Collins for long-winded conversations on craft, Andrew Newton for performative readings and getting hit on his bike (twice) and surviving (twice). Much love to Ricci Anselmi, may you rest in peace.

ABOUT THE AUTHOR

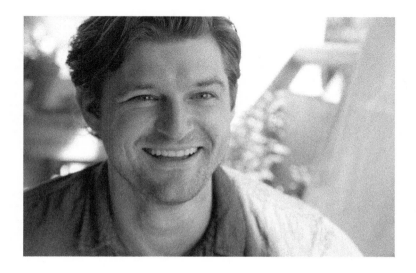

Kevin Bigley is an actor/writer from Yuba-Sutter County. He's most recently appeared in *Sirens, Bojack Horseman, Parked, Undone,* and *Upload.* He's had fiction published in *Maudlin House, X-Ray, Reedsy,* and *Beautiful Losers.* He lives in Los Angeles. Follow Kevin on Twitter @kevinbigley